# Dr. Gary A. Karl

# Dynamics of Back Pain

## *Helpful Hints to Becoming Pain-Free*

Teresa M. Karl, ed.
Photographs by Gary and Teresa Karl

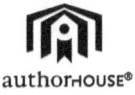

authorHOUSE®

*AuthorHouse™*
*1663 Liberty Drive, Suite 200*
*Bloomington, IN 47403*
*www.authorhouse.com*
*Phone: 1-800-839-8640*

*First published by AuthorHouse 12/18/2008*

*ISBN: 978-1-4389-1838-9 (sc)*

*Library of Congress Control Number: 2008910507*

*Printed in the United States of America*
*Bloomington, Indiana*

*This book is printed on acid-free paper.*

# Dedication

*To my wife Teresa,
whose encouragement and help has allowed me to accomplish
things I would never have imagined possible*

# Contents

# Contents

# Introduction

Over the years I've seen thousands of patients who complain of various types of back pain. Some involve the neck, while others involve the low back. Some affect the mechanics of the shoulder, while others affect walking and sitting. Some present as symptoms because of which patients have been made to feel foolish when nothing was found on testing to explain those symptoms. Some were caused by accidents, some by foolishness and stupidity. A large proportion, however, just happened. These patients cannot give you a good reason why it happened. They didn't lift; they didn't bend; they didn't overstretch; they didn't fall. It just happened. They made a quick turn, or sneezed, or turned over in bed. And there it was. The next question is, "Why did it happen to me and what are we going to do about it?"

Back pain has historically been an enigma to many physicians. They X-ray and scan hoping to find an answer that will satisfy the patient. They stick needles into the back to see if they can duplicate or alleviate the pain. They apply ice; they apply heat; they stretch the back with various modalities in the hope of relaxing those tight muscles; they prescribe medications to relax muscle spasm, to alleviate pain, and to relieve inflammation. And let's not forget surgical intervention for those difficult patients who constantly complain of pain and get no relief from these conservative therapies. Countless times during a new patient office visit have I had patients tell me their previous consulting surgeon prescribed their surgery without even examining them, basing that conclusion primarily on an MRI scan.

Unfortunately, that patient does not seek a second opinion, and undergoes the procedure the surgeon recommends. In some cases that patient recovers and does quite well. However, in my experience, this is not the scenario in most cases. Most patients end up with persistent pain, sometimes worse than that with which they started. They progress to undergoing multiple procedures, are prescribed high doses of narcotics to relieve pain, and may never be functional members of society again.

I've assisted surgeons with back surgery for 24 years. I have the greatest respect for good surgeons, and have been lucky throughout most of my career to have worked with talented orthopedic and neurosurgeons. It has been my experience that the better the surgeon, the less likely he or she is to rush in and do a surgical procedure. The only exception is in an emergency, which is rare. Good surgeons exhaust all the simple modalities first, to make sure that a surgical approach will get the best outcome for the patient. If a procedure is deemed necessary, the least amount of surgery to get the job done should be performed. Unfortunately, there are many surgeons throughout this country who do not share that opinion, and ultimately cause more harm than good. Their unfortunate patients must rely on care from pain management physicians for the rest of their lives. I have seen many patients who have undergone extensive and excessive procedures which might have been avoided if only common sense had been used in evaluating and treating them in the first place!

This book is written from a common sense approach. I will not quote statistics and lab data. This is not a text for training physicians. This is written for the patient who suffers back pain, and is confused as to what can be done and what direction he or she should take. Sometimes the simplest way is best!

# Chapter One
# The Nature of Pain

## Acute Pain

There are many formal definitions of pain. For most people, pain is an unpleasant sensation. If I hit my finger, with all my might, with a hammer, I will experience acute pain. A signal is sent from the receptors in my finger to my spinal cord. From there, a message will be sent from my spinal cord back to my hand. I'll probably pull my hand away and shake it vigorously. My finger will throb and swell. Blood vessels will rupture, fluid will flow into the traumatized soft tissue. Simultaneously, a signal will be sent from that level of my spinal cord to a higher level of my brain. Here the pain will be registered, and the sensation of severe pain will be felt at many levels of the brain. It will probably affect my speech areas causing me to shout obscenities for my stupidity! I may become nauseous, because the signal stimulated the vomiting center of the brain. It may trigger past experiences of similar pain in other areas in my brain. In a matter of milliseconds all these reactions have occurred, without conscious thought. Hopefully, I will now apply ice to my finger to keep it from swelling, and pray that I didn't fracture the bone. This is acute pain. Once the traumatized tissue stabilizes, the pain will disappear. Examples of acute pain include minor sports injuries, minor injuries sustained at home or at work, acute ruptured disc, sprains, and strains.

## Chronic Pain

Chronic pain is different. It starts out as acute pain. However, it sustains itself like a chain reaction once the cause of the acute pain has resolved. In this scenario, permanent changes occur in the spinal cord and levels of the brain over time. These affect various neurotransmitters throughout the nervous system. Patients have a difficult time recovering from chronic pain. The longer the chronic pain has been present, the more difficult it becomes for them to return to normal, if that is even possible.

Depression is a very common side effect of chronic pain. These patients are treated with a variety of medications including pain relievers, muscle relaxers, tranquilizers, antidepressants, neuroleptic agents and calcium channel modulating drugs. They undergo exhaustive testing including CT scans, MRIs, nerve conduction tests and discograms. They opt for epidural injections, spinal cord stimulators, and surgery. It is a challenge for them to regain functioning. Chronic pain patients include those suffering from fibromyalgia; chronic nerve pain as a complication of diabetes; chronic nerve irritation from a ruptured disc or spinal stenosis; postsurgical complications.

Acute pain may overlap chronic pain states.

## Combinations

Most patients that I have seen in practice fall between both categories. Many patients will suffer injuries and will wait days to weeks before seeking help. They thought they would get better on their own, but now can no longer tolerate the pain. Wishful thinking has passed. Some are now getting worried that they may have sustained a bigger injury than they originally thought. Some are forced to get examined because their spouses can no longer endure their constant moaning and groaning. Others can no longer perform their duties at work and are facing financial ruin. They have self-treated with miracle creams which are guaranteed to resolve pain, taken non-steroidal anti-inflammatory agents to relieve inflammation and stiffness, and tried an unending array of home remedies suggested by family members or friends. They have modified their way of walking, sitting, standing, or sleeping to alleviate the pain. It has become obvious to their family, friends, and employers that a problem exists. They are less productive at home or at work. They have searched the Internet for information and explanations for their pain. They find themselves trapped in a vicious cycle: they get little or no sleep, wake up tired and in pain, and expend a good part of their energy just to accomplish their daily functions and obligations.

Eventually they desperately seek the help of a physician or chiropractor. X-rays and scans are performed to ferret out the cause of their back pain. If some deformity is found in the spinal column, all attention, by both patient and doctor, is focused on devising ways to eradicate that problem. Unfortunately, most of the abnormalities that are seen on X-rays or MRI scans have nothing to do with causing the patient's original pain.

The most common cause of back pain is musculoskeletal in nature. It is a mechanical problem and is not necessarily seen on an X-ray or scan. It is determined by palpation, looking for the source of restriction of motion. The next most common cause that I have seen in my years of practice is ruptured disc, followed by degenerative arthritis/spinal stenosis/facet arthritis, and finally spinal cord tumors.

## Mechanisms of Back Pain

Yes, the majority of pain is muscular in nature! Receptors in the muscles constantly send back signals to the brain via the spinal cord and receive signals back in return. Small fibers in the muscles are constantly alternating in contraction/relaxation to create shape/tone. When all these fibers are stimulated at the same time, a muscle contraction occurs. Everything is in balance until a change occurs. When some sort of injury, insult, or accident occurs the brain sends out a massive number of signals to the various muscle groups to contract and protect more delicate, irreplaceable organ systems. Balance is disrupted. Muscles can stay in some contracted state indefinitely. This may occur for only a few days and resolve spontaneously. For example, you're working in the yard, and develop a sore neck or back over the weekend. By Monday you're good as new with a minimal amount of effort to recover. On the other hand, a whiplash injury which causes your neck to become rigid may not release for months.

Why this happens, no one knows for certain. Why would the body want to sustain such a counterproductive state? Is there an alteration in the signals from the receptors? Is the problem at the spinal cord segment? Is it that higher levels of the brain are affecting recovery? Is there a genetic component that may predispose a person to these problems? Perhaps it's a combination of all of the above.

Some researchers feel that in these cases, muscle receptors may start to send altered signals to the spinal cord saying that this new unbalanced state is normal. Thus, no attempts will be made by the nervous system to change or turn off the condition. Muscles contract and pull the spinal column to one side. The opposite groups of muscles are forced to be over-stretched. This will result in some pain, causing the patient to consciously try to correct the situation. This may involve a change in posture, leaning to one side, shifting weight. It may involve getting up and walking to stretch those tight muscles. Some patients will "crack their necks" or self-manipulate to get relief. Some will do some form of stretching for relief. However, in this chronic state, these measures offer only temporary relief and will not resolve the imbalance.

I have always taught medical students that if everything is in balance, there should be no pain or dysfunction. We have identical muscle groups on both sides of the body. When in balance, the muscle tensions are equal. There is no pain. There is no stiffness. When one side is in spasm, the muscle tensions change. This usually brings on some form of pain. Think of the example of a tug-of-war to explain this concept. If both sides are pulling equally, no side has the advantage. The people tugging on the rope go nowhere. If one side is pulling harder than the other, the strong side will have the advantage and will eventually win by exhausting their counterparts. The weaker side will try to pull harder but it will physically be impossible to win. They will end up being pulled to the opposite side. In spinal mechanics this leads to a restriction and loss of movement: stiffness and pain.

# Chapter Two

# The Causes of Back Pain

I have seen over the years that the causes of back pain seem to fall into four basic categories. The number one cause of back pain is musculoskeletal in nature. The second most common cause is herniated (ruptured) disc. Third is osteoarthritis/spinal stenosis/foraminal stenosis/facet arthritis. Fourth is spinal cord tumor. These categories apply primarily to patients who have not had previous back surgeries, congenital deformities, metastatic cancers, or infections. These are terms you probably have heard, but you may not fully understand their significance. Let's start with the least common and work our way to number one.

## Number Four: Spinal Cord Tumor

I have seen only three spinal cord tumors so far in my entire medical career, spanning thirty years. They are rare. Sometimes patients with chronic pain start to worry that they have a tumor. The odds are in your favor that you do not. The pain begins because the tumor is growing too large for the confines of the spinal canal in which it is located. It is usually gradual but severe pain which is usually out-of-proportion to physical finding. Diagnosis is confirmed with a CT scan or MRI. Treatment is surgical excision by a neurosurgeon. These tumors are usually not cancerous.

## Number Three: Osteoarthritis, Defined

Spinal stenosis, foraminal stenosis, and facet arthritis are usually the cause of osteoarthritis. Osteoarthritis is wear-and-tear arthritis. We all take for granted our skeleton, which is made up of bones connected together with ligaments. Joints form in between the connections to provide different types of motion: flexion/extension; internal/external rotation; adduction/abduction. Muscles attach to the bones to provide some form of locomotion around the joints. Bones are living tissues. They respond to different forces placed on them. If more force is applied, they will try to thicken to get stronger. If no force is applied, they get weaker and may start to lose density and mass. We tend to forget that as we age, our bones and joints also age. How many machines have you owned that after 30, 40, 50, 60, 70, 80 years or more still work? Even if your body doesn't work perfectly, it is still better than any machine manufactured by a human. So it is inevitable that with time, as your bones and joints age, the way you take care of those joints coupled with your genetic profile will dictate how much osteoarthritis you develop and how painful that osteoarthritis may become.

## Spinal Stenosis

The spine is made up of the spinal column (the backbone) which houses and protects the second component, the spinal cord. The spinal column is made up of many joints that are interconnected with the levels above and below each vertebra. The vertebrae themselves form a canal in which the spinal cord is protected and extends throughout your back to your skull. All these vertebrae are held together with strong ligaments in front and behind. The joints that connect the vertebrae actually allow movement. The spine can bend forward (flex), bend backward (extend), side bend to either side (lateral bending), and rotate to the right or left. This beautiful system allows the versatility of movement which we all take for granted.

In spinal stenosis, the canal in which the spinal cord is housed becomes narrower as the bones which make up the column thicken. This usually happens slowly over a period of time. As it does, eventually pressure is placed on the spinal cord. This brings about pain. Picture yourself in the middle of a comfortable room. Slowly the walls start moving inward. For a while you're okay, but ultimately if those walls don't stop moving in, you will be squished. That's spinal stenosis. Pain intensifies over time with movement and activity. Diagnosis is made with CT or MRI scans. Ultimately, if the causes for the stenosis aren't addressed, or if the patient lives long enough, extensive surgery will be required involving multiple levels of the spinal column. In many patients, however, pain can be brought under control with combinations of spinal manipulation, exercise/conditioning, and epidural injections.

## Foraminal Stenosis

Foraminal stenosis is similar to spinal stenosis, but it occurs in the space in the bone where the spinal nerves exit. It may be caused by a thickening of the bone. Many times it occurs because a herniated (ruptured) disc fragment is forced into the already tight space, making it even tighter. The nerve root becomes irritated and transmits nerve pain in relation to the spinal cord level. The pain may travel down an arm or leg. It may even present as pain from an internal organ. It can become very confusing especially because the nerves may not be "pure" from one spinal level, but may contain fibers from the level above and below as well. This is why it may be difficult to explain the exact pattern of pain to a physician and why it may take diagnostic testing to find the cause of the pain. This condition can also be brought under control with combinations of spinal manipulation, exercise/conditioning, and epidural injections. Surgery is an option if these conservative methods fail.

## Facet Arthritis

On the top and bottom edges of each vertebra is a cut (or "facet") defining the shape of the bone. These facets interlock with the ones on the vertebra above and the one below them. They actually are tiny joints, similar to the ones in your fingers and knees only much, much smaller. They are held together by ligaments. Their job is to limit and control motion in the spine. Sometimes these will become arthritic joints, and you may experience pain and stiffness with movement. If the ligaments which hold these joints together start to weaken, the vertebrae may start to move out of their normal position (a condition known as spondylosis). If many of these spots occur along the spinal column, surgery to stabilize the spine and prevent the spinal cord from compression may be required. However, most cases of facet arthritis are minimal and will stabilize if the conditions causing the back pain are brought under control. Spinal manipulation, exercise/conditioning, and epidural injections can accomplish this.

## Number 2: Herniated Disc

### Anatomy of a Disc

Herniated discs are another cause of back pain. This condition was unfortunately called "slipped discs" years ago, and I still hear that term occasionally from patients. Discs do not slip in and out. Picture a disc in your spinal column looking like a donut. The disc is composed of two regions: the outer ring portion (the dough) and a soft inner portion (the hole). The outer ring is made of fibrocartilage, and it provides support. Each vertebra is stacked on the disc below it and connected to the one above it. This fibrocartilage keeps each vertebra at the appropriate distance so that the spinal nerves may exit without being compressed. The inner portion of the disc is made of a softer material having the consistency of crab meat, and it acts as a shock absorber. It allows force from normal movement and support to be absorbed and dissipated (Figures 2.1, 2.2, 2.3). Imagine the vibration one would feel if these discs did not exist. It would be like driving a car without shocks or suspension on a bumpy road.

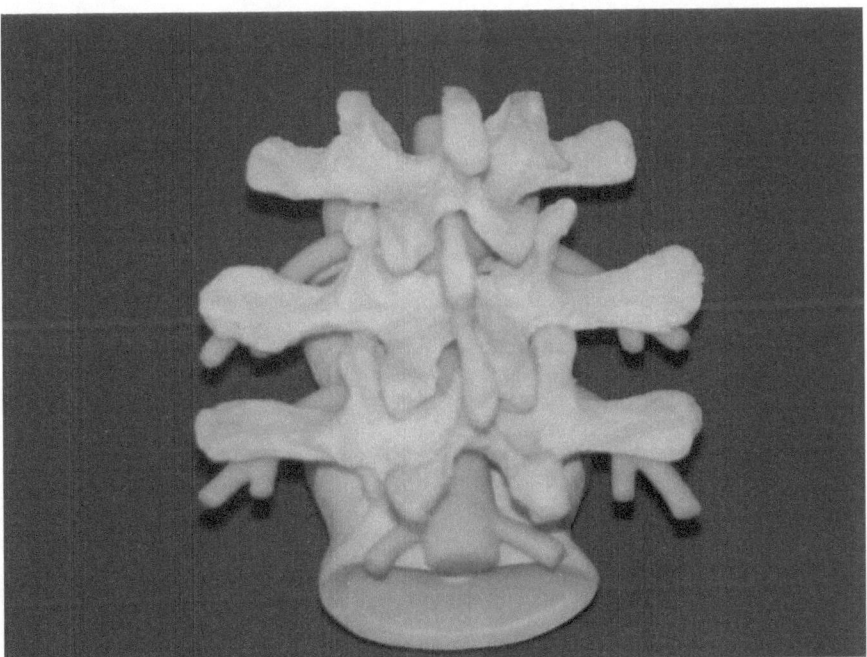

Figure 2.1   Normal Spinal Segment

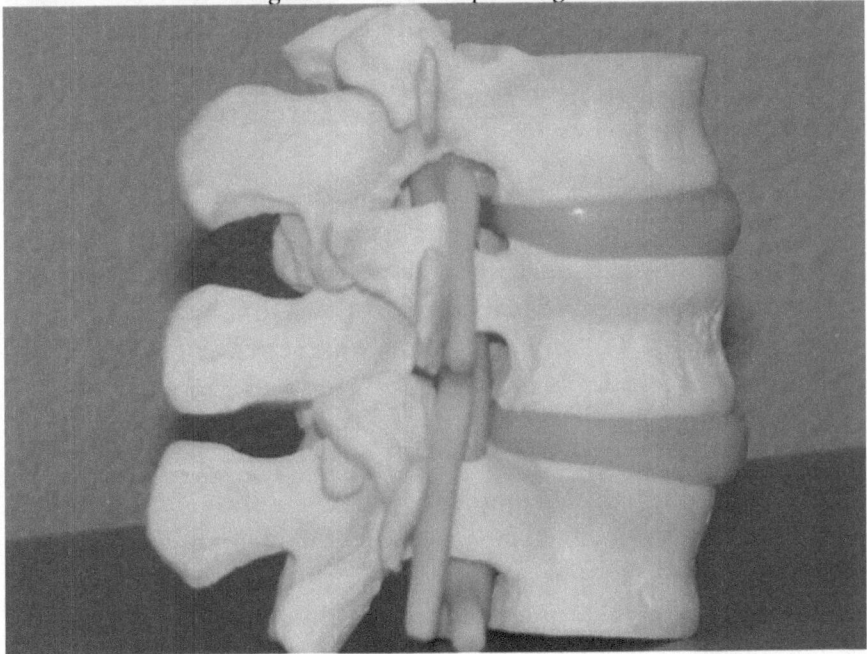

Figure 2.2   Side View Showing Discs

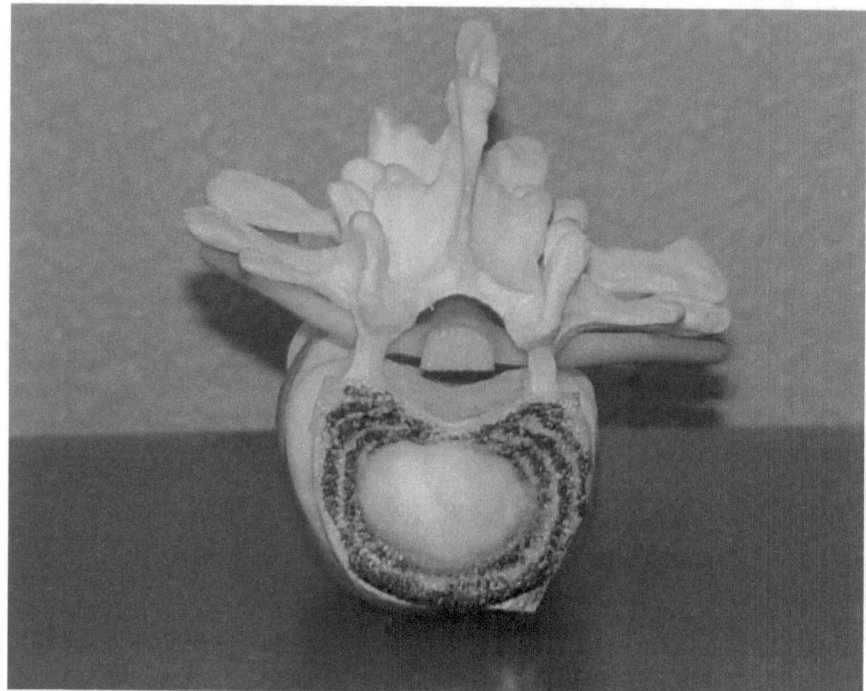

Figure 2.3   Normal Disc

## Factors Affecting Discs

The practice of walking upright coupled with the force of gravity causes the vertebrae to compress the discs over time, causing the discs to bulge. They lose water and dry out (dessicate) as they age. Like any part in a car's suspension, they eventually wear down to the point where two vertebrae come in contact with each other and can eventually fuse into one. This may lead to foraminal stenosis and nerve root entrapment, resulting in pain.

Many times the outer ring will tear or develop some type of hole, which under the right circumstances will allow the softer inner core to rupture into the spinal canal or neuroforamen. This is called a herniated disc. Sometimes the disc material cannot pass through the strong anterior spinal ligament to get into the spinal canal. This may be interpreted as a bulging disc on MRI or CT scan. What are the predisposing factors for this to happen? Genetics contributes to part of the problem. Some people have stronger discs than others. Age is another factor: if you live long enough, parts are eventually going to wear down. Activities throughout your life play a major role. People feel that they are indestructible! How many young adults are playing sports or engaging in recreational activities that they should avoid because they consistently get hurt? How many adults are working in occupations which they physically cannot handle? How many people have gone through training or some course designed to prevent injuries on the job and then ignore what they were taught? How many patients whom I have told how to avoid needing my services keep coming back because they don't listen?

## Rupture of Discs

Discs rupture when enough force at the right spinal column segment and the right time occurs as a patient bends forward or is flexed and twisted while moving forward. You can rupture a disc only with forward movement (flexion), not with backward movement (extension). The soft inner core is extruded from its confines within the disc (Figure 2.4),

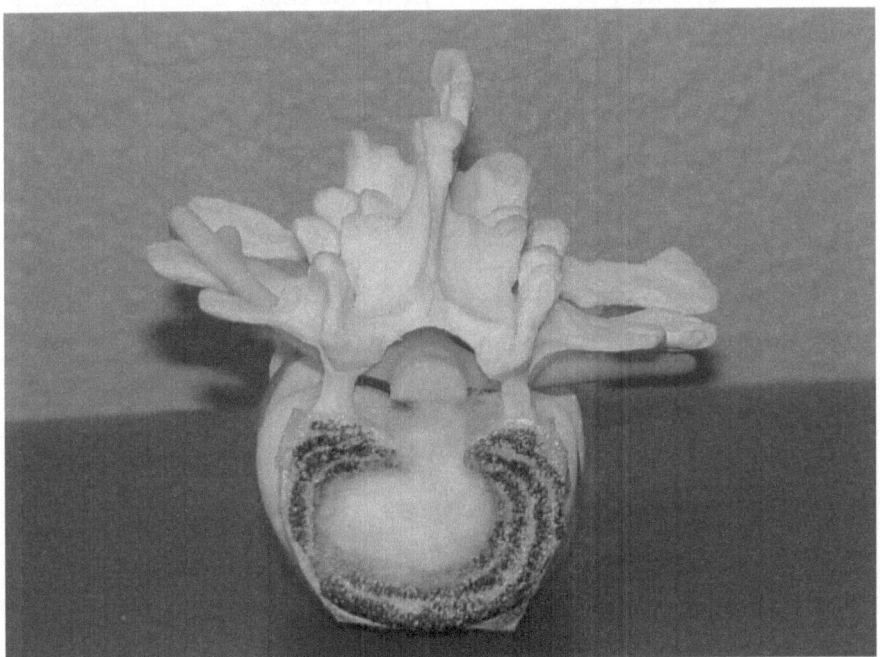

Figure 2.4   Ruptured Disc

sometimes bringing with it a small fragment of cartilage. When this material hits the spinal cord and/or nerve root, it will cause the cord or root to swell, transmitting pain. Imagine if someone came up to you and punched you in the shoulder as hard as he could. You would probably experience pain first, followed by some swelling of the muscles and tissues over the next few hours. If the injury is not severe, the pain will start to subside. If you're well-conditioned, it may subside very quickly. If you are poorly-conditioned, or if there are other chronic conditions present, it may take longer to go away. Eventually, if damage is minimal, the pain subsides.

Now, let's apply the analogy to the spinal cord. The disc is extruded forward toward the spinal cord or nerve. It hits these structures with considerable force. The covering around the spinal cord or nerve starts to swell. Signals are sent simultaneously to the higher areas of the brain. You feel pain! You consciously react, trying to assume a position which will relieve the pain. Signals are also sent out via the nerve roots to the muscles they innervate. These include the muscles down an arm or leg and the spinal muscles in the vicinity of the injury. The nerves down the arm or leg transmit pain.

In the leg, pain can extend down to the toes. In some cases, the pain may be felt in only part of the leg, perhaps only ankle pain, for instance, or just in the buttocks. The classic sciatic pain travels down the entire leg, from the buttocks to the foot. In the arm, it may present as shooting pain down the entire arm or forearm to the fingers. It may cause some numbness in some of the fingers. It may present as shoulder or shoulder blade pain that seems to never want to go away, or as soreness in the neck that won't resolve.

The other component involved in the ruptured disc is that signals are simultaneously sent to the muscles attached to the spinal column at the level of the injured nerve root. The muscles contract, or shorten, on themselves, because of the irritation.

Now check out the following diagram of a normal spinal column for a quick orientation in Anatomy of the Back 101.

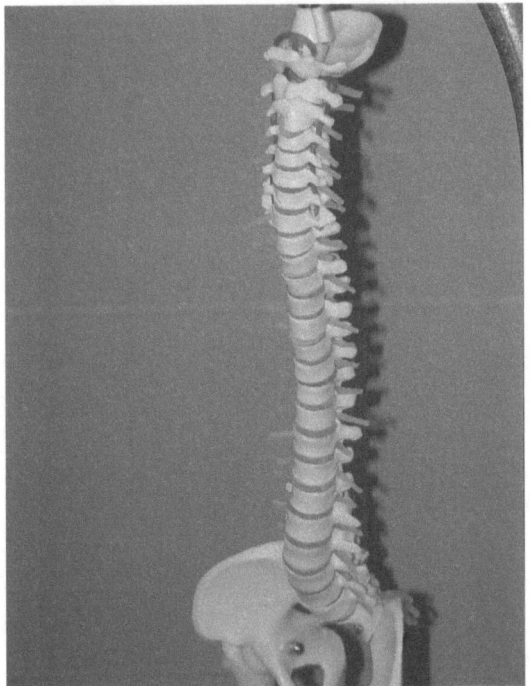

Figure 2.5   Normal Spinal Curves

In a normal back, the neck (Cervical Spine) and the low back (Lumbosacral Spine) have a curve opposite to the one in the middle back (Thoracic Spine). The cervical and lumbosacral curves are lordotic (the convex part of the curve faces forward) and the thoracic spine's curve is kyphotic (the convex part of the curve faces backward) (Figure 2.5). Can you guess why an early human spine evolved into ours? If the spine were absolutely straight from top to bottom, without the curves, all the weight of the spine plus everything attached to it would be transmitted down the entire length of the spine toward the sacroiliac joint (tailbone), pelvis, and legs. There would be tremendous forces placed on the lower lumbar spine and pelvis.

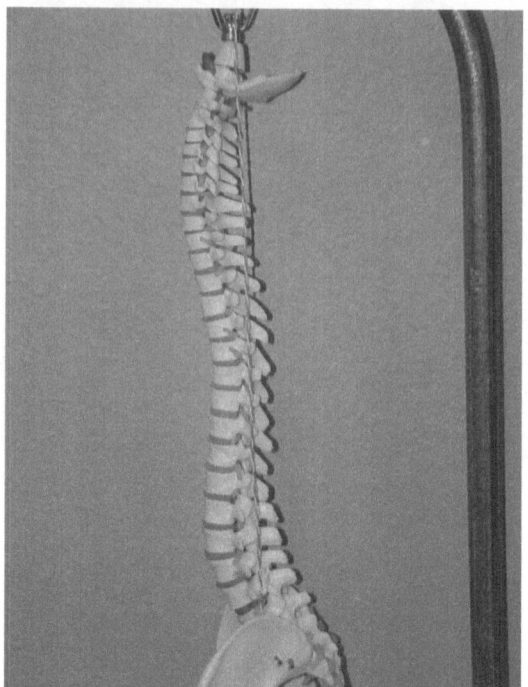

Figure 2.6   Plumb Line is Level!

Force is made up of horizontal and vertical components called vectors. The curves in the spine allow those vector forces at each vertebral level to be distributed over the curve, rather than straight down. Distributing the force evenly across all the spinal segments allows the spine to carry the weight more efficiently. It allows the spine to be balanced. If you drop a plumb line from the top of the cervical spine to the bottom of the lumbar spine, you will find it to be level (Figure 2.6). This allows the center of gravity to be concentrated over the spine, thus achieving balance.

It is this efficiency that is altered when the paraspinal muscles go into spasm after a disc ruptures. The muscles that cause problems most often seem to be the ones which attach to the front part of the spine in the cervical and in the lumbar areas. They contract, causing the normal curves to flatten. This redistributes the weight, further aggravating the injured spinal segment. Can you see how we are now back in that cycle of pain? The extra force near the rupture aggravates the nerve/spinal cord making the arm or leg pain worse. We respond by shifting our weight, standing and walking differently, tossing and turning in bed, all searching for that comfortable position in which all pain disappears. There occurs a constant tug-of-war between the right and left side of the body. Balance has been lost!

This can happen with you being unaware of it?

How did discs rupture in people who can't recall any trauma? Actually, there are probably many people who have ruptured discs and don't even realize it. Their discs had been wearing down because of age and repetitive trauma. This may include sitting at the computer with the head flexed forward, or habitually watching TV or reading in bed, or flexing forward when sneezing. They may have experienced pain for a few weeks and attributed it to "sleeping funny" or getting older. Whatever the case, the pain subsides and they do well. They develop no muscle weakness, loss of reflexes, numbness, or sciatica. The pain resolves spontaneously. Why were they so lucky?

Perhaps it was a small rupture. The herniated material may have had plenty of room to layer out in the spinal canal prevented further irritation to the spinal cord or nerve root. Maybe the patient identified the cause of the pain and changed behavior to prevent further rupture of the already herniated disc. Will that extruded disc material be absorbed? I have not seen this happen in clinical practice. Will it be sucked back into the disc itself and clear the spinal canal? I don't think this happens either, by itself or with the help of traction devices. Picture the herniated disc like a compressed tube of toothpaste. Pull off the cap and the toothpaste is extruded. Now try to put the toothpaste back into the tube without using your hands! That's how hard it would be to make a crabmeat-consistent material get back through a hole in the fibrocartilage of a disc.

Here lies the danger in making a diagnosis from an MRI or CT scan without thoroughly examining the patient and correlating their physical findings and history. Countless numbers of times have I seen a herniated disc on MRI which does not match the patient's symptoms and has nothing to do with his back pain.

## So, how do you know if you have a herniated disc?

Herniated discs represent a diagnosis in evolution. Very few patients in my practice have presented as the medical textbooks say they should. Leg pain or sciatica does not necessarily mean that you have a herniated disc. You can have leg pain and sciatica from other causes as well. The same is true of persistent excruciating neck or lower back pain. Numbness may be a result of muscle spasms or other metabolic diseases such as diabetes. Referred pain from other internal organ systems can mimic ruptured disc pain. It is a much more complicated diagnosis to make. So how is the diagnosis made?

There are patterns associated with ruptures which may not be obvious at first. Reflexes may be diminished, usually in the arm or leg which is experiencing the pain. Muscle weakness may be present on the herniated side in the affected extremity. Muscle weakness may also be present with pain caused by pure muscle spasm, but with no true loss of strength. In the case of ruptured disc with nerve involvement, there is true loss of muscle strength, and possibly atrophy (muscle wasting) if the condition has been present for a long time/if the initial trauma was severe. Your arm or leg pain may be aggravated by flexing, rotating, and side-bending into the area with the rupture, and it may be relieved by doing the opposite. The most intense muscle spasms can be felt on the same side as the herniated disc, rather than on the opposite side as in pure muscle spasms. There are additional leg-raising tests physicians can perform with you lying on your back to determine the source of pain.

## Treatments for Back Pain Caused by Herniated Discs

First-line treatment should include spinal manipulation to reduce muscle spasm, improve range of motion, and restore mechanical balance. This can be provided by an Osteopathic Physician (D.O.) or by a Chiropractic Physician (D.C.). I have found that trigger point injections into the muscles in spasm have also been helpful in reducing pain and spasticity.

Medications are not a cure for this problem; however, when used judiciously they will provide a means to help stabilize the patient more quickly. Anti-inflammatory agents play a role, if prescribed in dosages appropriate for the intensity of the problem. I prescribe prednisone (yes, the dreaded "steroid") when appropriate, over a 12-day period on a decreasing schedule. I find it allows the manipulated patient to suffer less muscle spasticity, which translates into less intense pain and better compliance in doing prescribed exercises and following other instructions. With decreased spasticity, I can achieve better movement with manipulation, restore normal range of motion, and speed up recovery. The correct muscle relaxer, chosen for the intensity of the condition as well as your response to such medication, can be a great help in reducing pain. Analgesics (pain-killers) play their role in helping reduce pain so that you can function with as near normal activity as possible, and allow you to sleep more comfortably. They should not be the main course of treatment! Everyone likes the quick fix, but it is very easy to become dependent on or addicted to these medications, especially when your pain has become chronic in nature. If narcotic pain relievers are prescribed for you, do not increase your dosage if the pain does not immediately subside without first consulting your physician. Do not see more than one prescribing physician. Do not accept medication from your friends or relatives which was prescribed for them when they had "a similar condition." Prescription drug abuse is fast becoming a nightmare in this country. Deaths occur from accidental overdoses and from combining incompatible drugs. Pain makes people desperate. Pain management is not and should never be synonymous with prescribing increasing doses of narcotics for pain control.

Other therapies include the use of ice packs to provide pain relief to the affected area. Application of heat is to be avoided, as although heat feels relaxing while it is being applied, it may increase muscle congestion and after a while will lead to more spasticity and increased pain. Extension exercises are helpful, as seen in Yoga or Pilates. All flexion is to be avoided! Physical therapy may be appropriate. Swimming is an excellent exercise. The water provides a medium of weightlessness and allows you to stretch more easily than if on land. It is important to stay as active as possible, but avoid all activities involving bouncing, jumping, and twisting.

Some patients find that they make improvement with the above therapies, and then level off just short of a return to normal. They seem to be excellent candidates for epidural injection at the spinal cord level which matches their remaining symptoms.

Of all cases of herniated discs I have encountered in my practices, 99% of them have resolved using the above treatments. There are only two reasons why I have ever recommended surgical intervention: if the patient has failed all the conservative measures we have tried, or if he has intractable pain along with loss of muscle strength and reflexes. If the above therapies are given sufficient time to work, all the patients who can recover will, leaving only the ones who truly need surgery. In the hands of a good, experienced surgeon, who is doing only what is absolutely necessary to relieve the patient's pain, that patient should have a good outcome.

## And Now, the Number One Cause of Back Pain

The most common cause of acute and chronic back pain, in both the upper and lower spine, is muscular in nature. Let me repeat that so that you can consider it carefully: the most common cause of acute and chronic back pain, in both the upper and lower spine, is muscular in nature. It is a mechanical problem which is multifaceted. There is probably a genetic predisposition to this problem: that is to say, it runs in families. The majority of patients interviewed over the years have had family members who have had some chronic back ailment. It could be their parents, siblings, grandma or grandpa, but someone had it or is being treated for it. We will devote the next few chapters to mechanical back problems in order to delineate their causes and treatments in full.

# Chapter Three

# Lower Back Pain

## What sets it off?

The trigger in low back pain usually involves some form of flexion at the waist or a combination twisting-flexion type movement. Examples are: lifting boxes from the floor; overstretching in the trunk of your car to pull out groceries; sit-up type exercises; slipping and falling down; falling from a height. There are probably thousands of ways to get hurt, but they do share some components. The initiating event can be simultaneous with the feeling of pain, but many times the patient reports that he or she did nothing to cause the pain. You may have only coughed or sneezed and suddenly felt severe pain. The initial cause of this lower back pain probably developed sometime in the 7-10 days prior to your feeling the severe pain. You initiated a low-grade spasm that was not painful—perhaps just some stiffness—nothing that you haven't experienced before. As you continued to perform your normal activities, spasms continued to increase slowly in intensity, just waiting for the right moment to become full-blown. At the right time, with the right movement, the lower back goes into full spasm. You experience severe pain throughout the entire low back extending into the tailbone or buttocks. If the sciatic nerve is involved, you may experience leg pain. The end result is immobility! You can't walk. If you can manage to get up, you are comfortable only when bending forward like a Neanderthal. Sitting becomes difficult. You start to shift weight away from the painful muscles in the hope of alleviating the pain. Getting up from your easy chair becomes impossible. You can't sleep because it is difficult to find a comfortable position. Even when you do fall asleep, turning over in bed causes more pain and wakes you up. After a few sleepless nights, you become exhausted, while the pain becomes even more intense. You take painkillers and muscle relaxers, anti-inflammatory agents, hot baths, but the pain never seems to go away. Sometimes it will wax and wane but it never quite goes away. Although some people may eventually recover on their own, you do not. After weeks to months of this suffering, depression may set in, complicating the original problem. You finally give in because this is now affecting your daily life and performance at work. You see your family doctor and are probably given more or different medications than you already have tried either by previous prescription or over the counter. These may have varying success. You're sent to physical therapy for six weeks in the hope of controlling these severe spasms. MRI scans will be ordered when this fails. But the MRIs show nothing at all! Everything is normal! Discograms will be ordered, looking for that elusive cause of the persistent back pain. Epidural injections will be discussed in the hope that this may alleviate the pain. You will be told that your back pain is due to your excessive weight, and once the weight is lost the pain should subside. When it does not, you will then be told to live with this condition. And all because your physician never actually palpated your back and felt the changes in the muscle tensions and range of motion which would have given him the greatest clue as to the cause of the pain.

### So what is the cause of this pain?

The mechanism for low back pain is similar to that seen in a case of herniated disc. The main difference is that there is no herniation of the disc. As the anterior muscles extending from the lower thoracic spine and along the entire lumbar spine go into extreme flexion, a flattening of the lumbar spine occurs, causing a redistribution of weight toward the tailbone. The pelvis shifts in response to this weight. It may rotate right or left. It may tip anteriorly (toward the front) or posteriorly (toward the back). The tailbone rotates, flexes, and locks into an abnormal position. The pelvis on one side may rise higher than the other side. Many times a combination of all these movements occurs. The ultimate result is your inability to walk, sit, and perform normal daily activities without pain. Various combinations of leg pain may develop depending on what nerve roots are irritated as they leave the spinal column and pass through these irritated spinal muscles. The muscle spasms and sciatic pain are usually on the opposite sides of each other compared to the pattern you would see with a herniated disc, in which case the sciatic pain and muscle spasm are usually on the same side.

## What to expect during the exam

The best and most appropriate way to treat low back pain is with spinal manipulation. This can be performed by an Osteopathic Physician (D.O.) or a Chiropractor (D.C.). I will limit my comments to Osteopathic Manipulative Treatment (OMT). Spinal manipulation is a physical process. It involves a hands-on approach which takes many years to learn, and a lifetime to try to perfect. Your medical history is extremely important as to how you injured yourself. There is always a cause, I need only ask enough questions to ascertain it. During this portion of the exam I closely observe you to assess the intensity of your pain as well as if secondary problems such as depression are setting in. This will affect treatment. What you say as well as how you say it has an importance. I will observe your posture: are you standing straight or do you lean to one side? Are you bent forward? Is one shoulder higher than the other? Is the spine normal or are there scoliotic curves? Does the pelvis appear level? Is there a leg length imbalance causing the pelvis to be unlevel? Do you move from a standing to a sitting position easily or with great difficulty, requiring more time to accomplish that maneuver? What is your age? Is this the first muscle spasm attack or one of many? Is there anything suspicious in your history involving other possible diseases which may be causing the back pain?

Palpating (feeling) the muscles along the spine gives a tremendous amount of information. Are the muscle tensions even? Are the muscles hard and ropey, or soft and swollen? Does the spine move equally in flexion, extension, rotation, and side-bending? As muscles go into spasm, motion is lost is the opposite direction of the muscle spasm. The muscles go into spasm and shorten on themselves, limiting rotation and side-bending to the opposite direction. Remember, you can always move more easily to the side of the muscle spasm than away from it. Is the motion at the sacrum or the tailbone altered? Has the pelvis shifted? All this information is necessary to determine what is actually happening in the spine, because treatment will involve doing the exact opposite! The search is for balance.

Finally, treatment techniques!

There are many forms of spinal manipulation. The point where the spine locks, or beyond which it will not move easily, is referred to as "the barrier." There are techniques in which a direct force pushes the spine past the barrier, restoring normal motion. Imagine a jar with a tight lid. Turning the lid, both on and off, should be easy and involve roughly an equal amount of force: the force to open the jar = the force to close the jar. Let's call this the normal range of motion for the jar lid. Now let's assume the cover is on extremely tight. As I turn the lid counterclockwise to open the jar, I encounter resistance (or a barrier). The lid does not want to come off easily. By approaching the barrier and applying more force, I get the lid off. I have restored normal range of motion to the lid. The normal range of motion in a human spine is restored by actually moving the vertebrae through a series of side-bending, extension, or flexion, and rotation past this barrier. Other techniques involve letting the muscles reset by moving the patient into the direction of the muscle spasm and holding him in this position until the muscles which are in spasm relax. The patient is then maneuvered back into normal position and range of motion manually. Some techniques involve relaxing the fascial planes of the muscles by direct stretching. Sometimes opposite groups of muscles are used to fatigue the ones in spasm, thereby restoring normal range of motion.

No matter what techniques or combinations thereof are performed, the end result should be re-establishment of normal range of motion and body mechanics. This is essential to controlling back pain. Education about why the muscles go into spasm and how to avoid such spasm in the future is also crucial.

## Do you need medication?

Anti-inflammatory agents and muscle relaxants have a role in trying to calm down these irritated muscles. There is no set combination of medications that works for every patient. The more difficult the patient is to manipulate and the more spasticity present in the muscles requires a stronger anti-inflammatory, such as prednisone, compared to a milder spasm which may respond to ibuprofen or naproxen. Muscle relaxants can be successful; however, the patient needs to be aware that the potential side effect is drowsiness. Ice pack therapy is effective for most patients. The only exceptions I have seen to this are those patients who have severe osteoarthritis or those who have some underlying collagen disease such as rheumatoid arthritis. They seem to do better with heat applications. Remember, if the therapy is going to work, it should have a long-lasting effect, not just a temporary one. You should feel better after treatment and not rebound into pain or spasm. For ice pack therapy, it is best to use a frozen reusable gelpack, not applied directly to the skin but with a towel or shirt in between.

## Heel lifts

For patients found to have a leg length imbalance, a heel lift which will level the pelvis is absolutely necessary to help alleviate low back pain. Patients with one leg shorter than the other will frequently mention that they felt better after manipulation for a few days, and then the pain returned. Correcting the short leg should alleviate this and also remove the constant feeling of tightness in the lower lumbar spine. This will be discussed in detail in an upcoming chapter.

## Posture while awake and asleep

Correct posture and exercise are extremely important in controlling low back pain. Muscle spasms in the lower lumbar spine will have a tendency to make you lean forward. This moves the center of gravity away from the spine and out of the body. Standing straight is extremely important, even if it is uncomfortable at the beginning of treatment. You cannot give in to the muscle spasms and expect to recover quickly.

You should use some type of support for the lower back while sitting or driving. This can be a lumbar support, small pillow, or even a rolled up sweater tucked behind the low back while sitting. This will extend the lumbar spine and force the muscles to relax. It will also help restore and maintain the normal curvature in the lower lumbar spine which had been altered by the muscle spasms. You should also avoid soft chairs which do not provide good support for the lower back. You have a tendency to flex forward while in a soft chair. This may increase muscle spasms, especially when you change position and try to stand up straight. A sudden change in position after sitting or driving for long periods of time may worsen the spasms. Getting up slowly and avoiding quick, sharp, jerky moves may help prevent further spasm and pain.

When sleeping, lying on your back or stomach will place more force on the lower lumbar spine and tailbone area, creating more pain. Lying on your side is a more neutral position. Do not sleep in the fetal position (knees drawn up and chin curled down to your chest)! This allows the flexor muscles in the low back to tighten, making it difficult for you to get out of bed and stand straight the next day.

## The value of exercise

Most patients do not wish to exercise when suffering muscle spasms, but it is extremely important to force the muscles to relax. Flexion-type exercises, such as sit-ups and touching your toes, are extremely popular, but will make the problem worse. They may even cause a disc in the lower lumbar spine to rupture or, in patients with osteopenia/osteoporosis, a fracture of a lumbar vertebra to occur. Extension exercises will help fatigue and stretch the anterior flexor muscles in the lower lumbar spine safely, even in high-risk patients with osteoporosis.

## Should you take Pain Relieving Drugs?

Analgesics play an important role in controlling the pain associated with acute severe muscle spasms in the lumbar spine. If you are in a condition of prolonged pain, you will not exercise, work, or be able to sleep. Sleep deprivation will aggravate your pain. This in turn will prompt you to take more analgesics. If you wake up exhausted and in pain, the day will go from bad to worse. You will be less productive. This will have a snowball effect, making each day worse, and leading to further muscle spasm due to inactivity and not exercising, and then greater use of analgesics. As time progresses, this may lead to depression. Analgesics are not, and never should be, the main treatment for back pain. Trying to control pain by increasing dosage accomplishes not a cure, but only a masking of the pain. Many narcotics are formulated with acetaminophen, which in itself can reach toxic levels and cause liver disease based on your overall health.

Narcotics are used frequently to control back pain. They are available in both short- and long-acting forms. There are different potencies based on the form of narcotic. Prolonged use of any narcotic may lead to tolerance of, dependence on, or addiction to the drug. In the acute phase of lower back pain, narcotics are valuable when they help provide sleep, and allow you to do your exercises and follow other recommended instructions. Within a reasonable amount of time, if there is no response to the primary therapies, further diagnostic testing is required to explain why the pain is still present, rather than just an increase in dosage of the narcotic. Treating the primary cause of the problem should eliminate the need for continuing analgesics, making abuse of these medications less likely.

The role of narcotics in treating chronic low back pain is a different story. These patients have had pain for months and possibly even years. Some may have had surgical intervention which did not solve the problem but antagonized it even more. Some have fibromyalgia, for which there is presently no definitive cure. Others may have severe degenerative changes which are impossible to prevent from progressing. Many of these patients need to be taking some form of analgesia daily. This group is at higher risk for developing dependence and addiction. These patients seem to fall into three categories.

The first type consists of people who have neither abused prescribed medications nor experimented with illegal drugs and are now caught in a state of panic. They're frustrated that they are not able to perform their normal daily activities, and may be depressed. They have tried many different medical and surgical regimens, and all have failed. Their quality of life has deteriorated. Analgesics may restore some of that quality of life for this type of patient, who will use the lowest dosage necessary to control the pain to avoid becoming tolerant or addicted. Some of these patients even take a sub-therapeutic amount to avoid addiction. These patients are least likely to become abusers of narcotics.

The second group of patients has chronic pain because of their occupations. They get some relief from treating the main cause of their problem; however, their daily activities exacerbate the problem over and over again. They usually cannot take any time off from work to adequately recover. They report that their symptoms do subside when they eventually have a vacation. They tend to be more compliant and reliable patients. They try to keep their analgesic use at the prescribed levels, for both short- and long-acting drugs. They tend to increase their usage only if they get an extreme flare-up of back pain and feel they can get it under control within a few days. These patients don't ask to escalate the potency of their medications, or, if they do it's only for a short period of time until they're back to normal. They may develop a degree of dependency on the medication over time but do not seem to become addicted to it.

The third type of patient may have a history of drug experimentation in his youth, or have a tendency to be an alcohol abuser. These are the patients who escalate the dosage of their medications without consulting their physician. They may run out of their medications earlier than expected, and return sooner for follow-up visits than what was scheduled. They complain that the lower potency analgesics are ineffective, and try to steer the physician into ordering more potent ones. They try to make the physician believe that there is no way they will become addicted to these drugs, and that they need these medications to perform their normal daily activities at home and at work. These patients are less compliant to following directions. Many are in denial that these meds are affecting their daily performance. Rather than trying to resolve their underlying problems, their main concern is continuing their analgesic usage. These patients do very poorly. They have a high predilection for dependence, addiction, and depression. They are at a high risk for overdose and death. They need to be treated in a substance-abuse center for detoxification and rehabilitation.

## The role of anesthesia in treatment

Anesthesiologists are a very important adjunct to manipulative medicine. They can achieve especially beneficial results for patients who suffer lower back pain from herniated disc or have components of facet arthritis which has partially improved with manipulation but are still experiencing pain, or seem to flare up with minimal activity. Epidural injections have benefit if there is a target at which the anesthesiologist can aim. They do not seem to be effective in patients who have normal anatomy as seen on MRI.

Some chronic pain patients who have failed all other conservative approaches may benefit from catheters infusing medication directly into the spine via a small pump. These are not without complications. Present literature shows that these pumps may ultimately cause problems over long-term usage. The majority of back pain can be controlled with the use of manipulation, anti-inflammatory agents, muscle relaxants, analgesics, exercise/posture, and epidural/facet injections. Less than 1% of the patients in my practice ever need surgical intervention.

## So, should you have surgery?

Surgical intervention is necessary for a select few patients. The majority of back pain is not caused by a problem which can be corrected by surgery, although I'm sure many surgeons will disagree. Patients who are surgical candidates are those with a herniated disc which did not respond to manipulative therapy, epidural injection, and other conservative therapy. Spinal cord tumors and significant spondylolithesis with spinal cord and nerve root compression also require surgery. Years ago, before epidural injections were routinely performed, I would send approximately fifty patients per year for lower back surgery to decompress a nerve root from a herniated disc. After epidurals became more widely available, that number dropped to less than five per year. I feel that the number of back surgeries performed in the United States each year is excessive.

Too many patients undergo disc fusions. More and more articles lately are questioning the sense of performing these procedures for low back pain, since many of them do not alleviate the original pain and actually may make it worse. This may lead to multiple surgeries being performed on the unfortunate patient in the hopes that the next procedure will ultimately solve the problem. Of course, if the procedures fail, the patient will suffer chronic pain and will most likely need to rely on narcotics for the rest of his life. Fusion of selected segments of the spinal column may destabilize other areas over time, since both normal anatomy and normal mechanics have been altered.

There is a place for back surgery; however, with the exception of a life-threatening spinal cord injury or spinal cord tumor, it is not the first choice. Good surgeons will try all conservative measures first before contemplating surgery. They do not base their surgical decisions on MRI scans alone, but correlate them with the patient's history and physical findings. Many times I've seen surgeons order more invasive testing to justify doing a more complicated surgical procedure, such as a spinal fusion, when microsurgery to decompress an entrapped spinal nerve root may have been all that was necessary to solve the problem. Get a second opinion before undergoing any aggressive surgical intervention to your lumbar spine.

# Chapter Four
# Upper Back Pain

Upper back pain is very similar to what has been described with lower back pain in regard to the mechanisms which cause it. Most patients will complain of pain in the neck, upper back, or shoulder regions. Some may present with chronic headache or jaw pain. Some will complain of weakness in the arms or numbness/tingling travelling down their arms into the hands. They feel as if they have lost strength, especially when lifting or gripping objects. These problems can occur with normal daily activities, or may be the result of some type of accident. Many patients have no idea what brought on the problem. Some patients will attribute it to "sleeping funny," being out of good physical shape, or just getting older. There's usually a significant loss of normal range of motion in the neck; however, it may have occurred over such a long period of time that the patient does not truly notice it and thinks it's a normal aging process.

## Anatomy of the Upper Back

Seven vertebrae make up the cervical spine. The spinal cord travels from the brain through these seven vertebrae to connect with the thoracic spine. The vertebrae are somewhat smaller than those seen in the lower lumbar spine. This causes the spinal canal (which houses the spinal cord) and neuroforamen (where the nerves leave the spinal cord) to be proportionately smaller compared to the lower back. Bulging or herniated discs may have more significance in this smaller space. The curvature in the neck is similar to that seen in the lower spine. It is lordotic (curves forward) in nature. The neck is surrounded by strong muscles which allow flexion (forward bending), extension (backward bending), side-bending, and rotation. Many of these muscles attach to the upper back, shoulders, and upper chest. The nerve supply leaving these vertebrae pass through columns of muscles as individual nerves until they reach the axilla (armpit) where they intertwine and create the final nerves which extend down into the arm.

## So, what is the cause of the Pain?

Triggering off upper back pain usually involves some form of flexion in the neck. This may be from chronic forward bending at work, hobbies, sitting at a computer, knitting or crocheting, twisting while playing a sport, sleeping with the head flexed too much instead of in a neutral position, falling asleep while watching television, reading propped up with pillows, and so on. It can involve severe instantaneous muscle spasm as seen in a whiplash-type injury from an automobile accident or sports injury.

Whatever is the initiating event, flexion is involved. The muscles in the front of the neck will tighten, causing some straightening of the cervical vertebrae. This will sometimes cause a "flattening" of the cervical spine seen on X-ray. The muscles in the back of the neck will tighten to compensate. The force is usually most intense at the base of the skull which attaches to the spinal column, and at the base of the neck. Some patients complain of pain from the skull down to the shoulders. As the spasms extend into the thoracic spine (chest), there is a tendency for the muscles to pull down on the shoulder blades, causing a loss of normal motion in the shoulder. It becomes more difficult to raise your arm over your head, comb or brush your hair, put on a shirt or blouse, or do any type of exercise which involves abduction (moving your arm away from your body) of the shoulder.

These muscle spasms disrupt the normal balance in the neck, causing your head to feel extremely heavy and difficult to support. Some patients even say it's impossible for them to lift their heads up from a pillow after sleeping. The head feels like a giant bowling ball! They have to use their hands to help support the head on the neck. Their center of gravity has been disrupted by muscle spasm. Many patients also experience numbness or tingling down the arms with these muscles spasms, because the nerve and blood supply to the arms pass through the columns of muscle. When those muscles go into spasm, they act like a vise putting pressure on the vessels and nerves. This can cause anything from a sensation of shooting pain to the fingertip, to numbness or tingling down the arms, to feeling a loss of grip strength even though no strength is truly lost. Prolonged neck spasm may cause muscle tension headaches, and may bring about or aggravate temporomandibular joint (jaw) pain.

## Treatment Techniques

Treatment for the spasms depends on their intensity. The most important thing to remember is that range of motion should be restored as soon as possible to prevent chronic pain from developing. This can be achieved through manipulative treatments performed by osteopathic physicians or by chiropractic physicians. There is a wide range of techniques which can be performed, depending on the patient and on the skill of the practitioner:

- Soft tissue techniques which involve stretching and slowly articulating the spine are very effective in patients with severe muscle spasm or osteoarthritis.
- Fascial release techniques are a form of stretching against the grain of the muscle in the area of most intense spasm, which causes it to release and relax.
- Counterstrain techniques can be performed by gently moving the patient into a position of balance, relieving the pain and muscle spasm, then gently moving him into normal position.
- Muscle energy techniques use the opposite group of muscles to fatigue the ones which are in spasm, which promotes relaxation and restoration of normal range of motion.

Non-manipulative treatments are also valuable in the quest for restoration of normal range of motion and alleviation of upper back pain. Trigger point injections into the most reactive part of the muscle in spasm may provide relief. Regarding medications, a short course of cortisone may be appropriate to relieve inflammation in the patient who just sustained a severe whiplash or sports injury. I've found that in extremely stiff patients who are in a great deal of pain, a combination of prednisone and Valium is very effective in reducing muscle spasm. In patients with less spasticity, an anti-inflammatory and analgesic may be all that is necessary. Muscle relaxers play a role in improving range of motion in the neck. These drugs are not my first line of treatment, since they cause drowsiness and may affect performance while driving or working heavy machinery. Analgesics may be used to enable sleep and allow performance of normal activities throughout the day at home and at work. Again, medications are not the main treatment. Sometimes, patients who obtain relief using a narcotic pain reliever feel that it is the cure for their problem. Warning: Narcotics mask pain. They do nothing to alleviate the muscle spasticity, correct the mechanical deficits, or relieve inflammation. They are temporary measures to help stabilize you enough to allow you to do what you need to do to get better. These drugs are potent, and are prone to cause dependence which can lead to abuse over time.

## Should you curtail your activities?

On the contrary! It is extremely important to keep as active and as close to your normal routine as possible. Disrupting your routine at home and at work will cause you more difficulty in getting back to normal. Inactivity will make you stiffer. Increased muscle stiffness will cause you to be less active, leading to more pain and stiffness. Around and around the cycle goes. This sets you up for chronic back pain, depression, and disability.

Rather than curtail activities, some simple rules should be kept in mind when performing normal daily activities. Good posture is extremely important. If you have severe neck spasms, you must avoid constant flexion at the neck. That is, do not do anything that will cause you to keep your head bent forward. The rules:

- Do not watch television or read while lying on your side with your head propped up on your arm.
- Do not use more than one pillow while sleeping, to avoid pushing your head into extreme flexion or side-bending throughout the night.

- Sit up straight while working at your computer. Your workstation should be adjusted so that your monitor is at eye level. Sit in a comfortable chair with a small pillow for support in the area of the lumbar spine which will allow you to sit more erect.
- Never bend your head to your shoulder to support a telephone. If you need to be on the phone constantly, a headset or Bluetooth system should be incorporated into your routine.
- Any activity which involves working with your arms over your head should be kept to a minimum.
- Multiple short breaks/stretches will help prevent your neck muscles from going into full spasm if taken periodically throughout your work day.

## Exercise Recommendations

Exercise is extremely important. People with sore necks avoid moving their heads because of the pain or the fear that they might cause more damage. Gentle range of motion exercises, with forward, backward, side-bending and rotation are a powerful way to restore normal mechanics. Here is one I recommend to my patients:

1. Roll up a towel to a 2- to 3-inch diameter thickness (Figure 4.1).

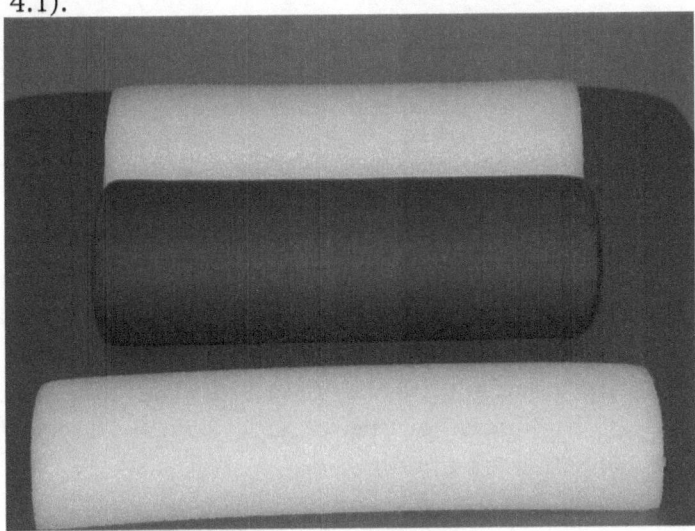

Figure 4.1  Towel Rolls

2.  Lie on the floor on your back.
3.  Place the towel roll across your spine behind your shoulder blades to stretch your upper back and neck muscles (Figure 4.2).

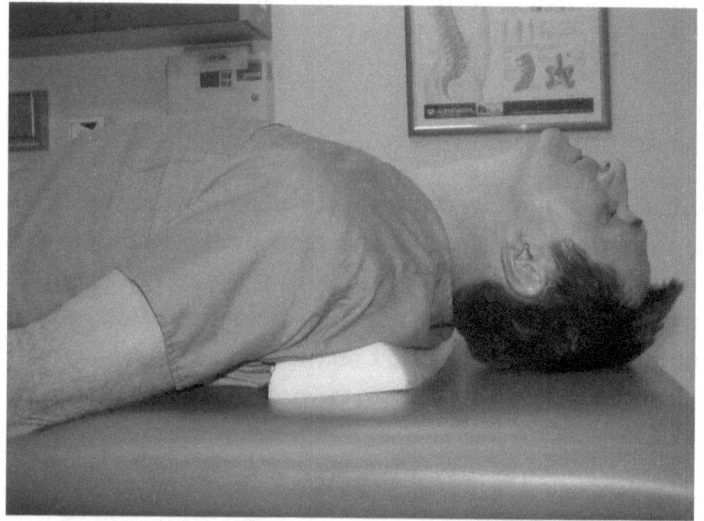

Figure 4.2   Roll placed behind Shoulder Blades

4.  Do this for a few minutes at a time, periodically throughout the day to prevent stiffness and relieve spasm.
5.  If you have flattening of the cervical spine, place a smaller towel roll directly under your neck and let your head gently extend for a few minutes at a time   (Figure 4.3).

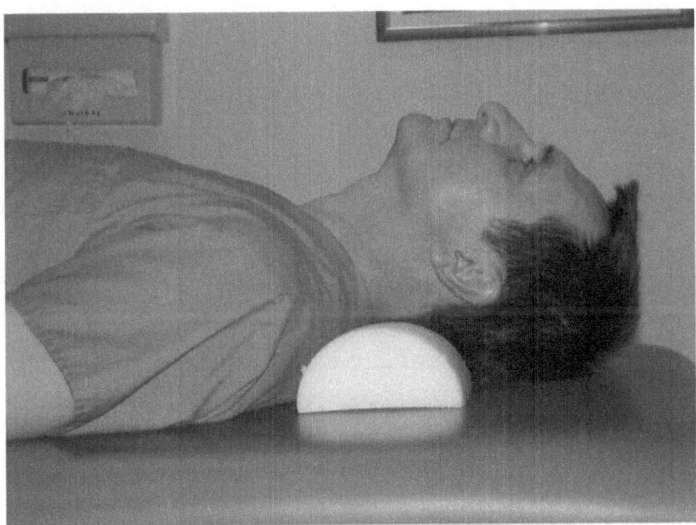

Figure 4.3   Roll placed under Neck

## Ice Packs vs Heating Pads

Application of icepacks to your neck, upper back, and shoulders will decrease inflammation, relieve pain, and in the long run help you achieve normal range of motion faster than with applications of heat. Heat and whirlpool treatments have a tendency to give temporary relief; however, in the long run, they antagonize the muscles and make them stiffer. Remember, heat increases blood flow into tissues/muscles that have already been irritated by some force. These tissues become more congested. The muscles that are in spasm now become "waterlogged" and usually respond by tightening even more. This is interpreted by the patient to mean that the heat "wore off" and the muscles got tighter, rather than that the heat aggravated the muscles which were already irritated, and they became tighter. The only exceptions I've seen to this are patients with underlying collagen diseases such as rheumatoid arthritis or severe degenerative arthritis. In those patients heat may be more beneficial than ice because of the underlying arthritic disorder.

## Concomitant Therapies

Massage therapy, physical therapy, acupuncture, and Pilates/Yoga all have a role in helping restore normal mechanics in the neck and upper back. Physical therapy is especially appropriate in patients who lack the motivation to exercise at home, are disabled, or who are not very compliant in following instructions. Physical therapists can reinforce and continue the team effort to try to get these patients under good control.

Epidural injections are not successful in treating neck pain caused by muscle spasm unless herniated disc, spinal stenosis, foraminal stenosis or facet arthritis is present.

## Neck Pain from Causes Other Than Flexion

A herniated (ruptured) disc or spinal stenosis may present similarly to pure muscular pain. All three can cause severe neck pain, muscle spasms, and loss of normal range of motion in the neck, upper back, and shoulders. They can involve arm pain, numbness, or tingling. They may contribute to muscle tension headaches. They may refer pain to the shoulders and mimic a shoulder problem. These entities are usually found when the patient fails to respond to conservative therapies mentioned previously.

## What tests are needed?

X-rays have little value in assessing for a ruptured disc, spinal stenosis, or nerve root entrapment in the intervertebral foramen. An MRI scan of the cervical spine will reveal these problems. Again, this test is not ordered on first evaluation unless there is something in your history that is extremely suspicious, requiring such a scan. Focusing on the scan too early in the evaluation may make the physician miss the original cause of your pain. Many people have abnormalities in the cervical spine without suffering symptoms. If you fail conservative therapy and are doing everything possible to alleviate the spasm without the desired result, then an MRI scan should be ordered. If the pathology seen on the MRI scan matches the physical findings, then that pathology is probably part of the cause of your pain. Other components of your pain are the muscle groups attached to the spine which are innervated by the nerve roots irritated by that spinal pathology.

Discograms are test procedures in which a needle is carefully inserted into an intervertebral disc. Contrast dye is injected into the disc under pressure in the hopes of reproducing your pain patterns. If your pain can be produced with the injection, it is considered a positive test and the disc is "diseased." This procedure is carried out on each cervical disc. This procedure should not be considered routine for patients with neck pain. It is done increasingly more often in patients who complain of pain yet have a relatively normal MRI scan of the neck. It has some value in those particular cases, but is still considered experimental by insurance companies who deny benefits for it.

## Treatments

Epidural injections, given by experienced anesthesiologists, can help to alleviate pain indefinitely from a herniated cervical disc, mild spinal stenosis, and mild intervertebral foraminal stenosis. A common complaint that I have heard constantly from patients is that the epidural injections just mask pain. In reality, these injections deliver cortisone and a long-acting analgesic to the site/sites in question using a fluoroscope. The purpose is to alleviate pain by decreasing swelling of either the spinal cord or the nerve roots which are causing the pain and suffering. They are usually given in a series of three injections a week or two apart. I have found that if the patient does not respond by the second injection, a third is probably not going to be effective. Their effects may be long-lasting when combined with lifestyle modification, good posture, manipulative treatments, exercise, and so on. A program of epidural injections along with spinal manipulation has allowed 99% of my patients to become stable and not require surgery.

For those patients who have failed conservative therapy and have a definitive pathological spinal lesion which can be seen on MRI and is causing the problem, surgery may be the ultimate therapy to alleviate that pain. The least aggressive surgery to get the job done is the one that should be performed.

# Chapter Five

# Unequal Leg Lengths:
# The Short Leg Syndrome

I have noticed over the years that many patients who suffer from back pain have characteristics in common. This holds true across all age levels, from teens through 20- and 30-somethings through 40-50-60-year-olds. The complaints range from persistent "migraine" headaches (which are really muscle tension headaches) to jaw pain, to tightness in the neck/shoulders/between the shoulder blades, to low back pain, to hip or knee pain. They may have no history of injury. If they have been injured, recovery took a long time, or indeed has still not been accomplished. All have persistent pain, including some feeling of tightness even on a day they feel is good. They seem to be more prone to flare-ups of back pain compared to other people in similar circumstances, age, and health. Family histories usually reveal that either one or both parents or siblings also suffer persistent pain. X-rays, CT/MRI and brain scans are negative for pathology. Massage therapy seems to give them temporary relief for an average of three days before the pain starts again. Physical therapy modalities such as high voltage muscle stimulation will give temporary relief, with patients reporting that their pain is back by the time they leave the office or shortly thereafter.

These are all characteristics of patients who have unequal leg lengths: one leg is shorter, often by only a few millimeters, than the other.

## The Importance of Equal Leg Lengths

People are not perfectly bilaterally symmetrical. When measuring leg lengths years ago using a computer-assisted device called a Metricom,

I was surprised to find how often bones were not of equal length. Many times the total length of the right leg (hip to ankle) would equal the total length of the left leg (hip to ankle), even though the measurement of the right leg (hip to knee) would be shorter than the left (hip to knee) , because the right (knee to ankle) would be longer than the left (knee to ankle).

Why is this important? Let's use a house as an example. The foundation of the house is composed of footings to support beams and the walls to support the frame of the house. The idea is to take all the weight and spread that force across the structures for support. Otherwise, the house would fall down. The foundation balances and supports the entire weight of the house and all of its contents. It provides stability and strength to the structure. Great care is taken to make sure that the foundation is absolutely level. If it is not, the structure will experience shearing forces which will make it unsound and weak. Walls and ceilings will crack. The house will not remain plumb.

How does this apply to your body? The pelvis (foundation) supports all the weight of the body and its parts. We have seen that the various curves throughout the spinal column allow force to be dispersed throughout its entire length to prevent excessive force in the pelvis. When your leg lengths are equal, a plumb line drawn from the skull to the sacrum (tailbone) should be perfectly straight, allowing the most efficient balance and weight distribution throughout the entire spine.

Now, let's suppose that your left leg is shorter than your right leg. Your pelvis will tip slightly to the left. Your spine will still try to be perpendicular to the pelvis, however, that will make you walk crooked. To compensate and keep balance, your spine will gently roll to the right. The muscle tensions in your lower lumbar spine are no longer equal. The muscles on the short-legged side have a tendency to be dominant, and will predispose you to more muscle spasms on that side. Truly, all back pain is not caused by a short leg alone; however, the short leg will prolong the muscle spasms unless the imbalance is corrected. Over time, the imbalance is transmitted up to the shoulders, neck, and head, contributing to muscle tension headaches and even jaw problems.

This is easy to see if we use the example of a tile floor. Those of you who have laid ceramic tile will know exactly what I am talking about. For those of you who have not had the pleasure, you'll have to take my word for it. If the first tile laid is not perfectly straight (plumb), each ensuing tile will be slightly off. It won't seem like much until you reach the last tile. Then you will see a marked deviation from a straight line. The farther you move from the origin, the worse the defect becomes.

In the body, the farthest away from the pelvis is the neck/head. When I was a first-year medical student, I had the pleasure of listening to a lecture on Temporomandibular Joint (TMJ) Syndrome given by the chairman of the Oral Surgery Department. I remember him saying "TMJ Syndrome, look for a short leg." I thought he was absolutely crazy! How does a short leg cause jaw problems? Now when I ask patients who have unequal leg lengths if they have also experienced jaw problems, they are flabbergasted. How did I know they were having problems up there when they came in complaining of lower back or neck pain? I no longer consider the lecturer to be crazy. I appreciate his having informed us of that relationship. It definitely has affected the way that I approach and treat these problems.

Persistent tension headaches, especially in young adults/children with negative neurological workups, have also been associated with short leg syndrome that has gone unnoticed and untreated. I have found in my present population of patients that sometimes migraine headaches are being precipitated by muscle tension headaches associated with a short leg. Correct for the discrepancy in leg lengths with a heel lift of the correct thickness worn in the shoe on the short leg side, manipulate the spine, and use whatever modality you choose to relieve pain and spasticity, and most patients get better.

## It's off by *how* much?

Unfortunately, many practitioners, D.O., M.D., and chiropractors alike, either don't realize that a short leg is present, feel that they can lengthen it with manipulation, or think that it really doesn't matter. If the leg is truly short, it will not get longer with manipulation no matter how hard or long you try. Sometimes a patient exhibits a relatively short leg due to muscle spasms in the pelvis. If the muscle spasms can be eliminated, the leg lengths will become equal in these patients. But that just means they never had a truly short leg.

Most orthopedic surgeons look at small discrepancies (millimeters) in leg lengths as not significant. I would periodically have this discussion with a very good friend of mine who is an orthopedic surgeon in Chicago. My comeback to him would always be, "Go home and cut two opposite legs of your wife's coffee-table off by an eighth of an inch and tell me how she feels about that." Then I would get this look from him that said, "Smart ass!" You know what would happen to that table with unequal leg lengths: glasses would tip to one side. Objects that could roll would, right off the table. This small discrepancy is not acceptable in a piece of furniture. Why should it be acceptable in any human being? When the pelvis is not level, everything supported by the pelvis is tipped to one side. The body contorts itself to balance the condition. Instead of equal muscle tensions, opposite groups of muscles will be put under more tension. This requires work to accomplish and energy to maintain. It is no surprise that patients with chronic back pain associated with short leg syndrome will feel better in the morning after rest and start to get their worst pain later in the afternoon when they get tired. Add to this the fact that people are lifting, bending, twisting, running, climbing, and so on, and you can see how a small and "insignificant" discrepancy may ultimately lead to larger problems. How many patients develop recurrent back pain which ultimately leads to surgical intervention because no other therapy worked? There are many patients presently in my practice who despite having had surgical interventions in the past based on chronic back pain and MRI findings still have back pain because their short leg syndromes have never been addressed. How many of these patients would have obtained relief with conservative therapy and could have avoided surgery? Even now, correcting for leg length discrepancy will bring them some relief, but not at the level that might have been achieved prior to the surgical intervention which has further distorted their anatomy.

## You Had the Wrong Parents!

Short Leg Syndrome runs in families. I am sure there is a genetic predisposition for this problem. I don't feel it occurs at random. I inherited mine from my mother. My youngest son inherited his from me. Surprisingly, most short legs I have seen are on the left side. I have no idea why this is so, because the right leg is affected in my family line. Most likely, discrepancies probably occur during rapid growth spurts in young children, so it is important to start screening children for short leg syndrome. I counsel families in which one member has a short leg that any future member is at risk for developing one. If your pediatrician tells you that your child has a mild curvature in the back which does not appear to be significant, examine leg lengths. If they are unequal, level the pelvis using a heel lift to compensate for the difference. This would be analogous to a young tree sapling starting to grow crooked. If the tree were starting to tip to one side, it would be straightened by staking it to the opposite side with cable. Keeping the tree in this position as it continues to grow usually results in a tree with a straight trunk. The same can occur with children. Leveling the pelvis at a young age should straighten the spine. This method worked on my son. He wore a heel lift in his shoe during his formative years. His adult spine is straight and he is much taller than I! There was a study years ago in the Journal of the American Osteopathic Association that found correcting for the short leg could straighten the spine in adults, but no mention was made of the pediatric age group at that time. From my experience, leveling the pelvis in adults has not really corrected the mild scoliotic curve in their backs even though it helps alleviate their back pain. Earlier intervention, I feel, has a better chance of allowing the spine to remain straight while growth occurs, and so avoiding any extraneous curves. Also, patients with scoliosis who have had corrective surgery may afterward have a short leg contributing to their pain postoperatively.

## You had the Wrong Surgeon!

There is a new group of patients who were neither born with nor developed a short leg during their lifetime, but now have one because of joint replacement surgery. Orthotic devices (knees, hips, ankles) come in various sizes. The surgeon must be cognizant and careful to avoid creating a short leg after installing a total hip or total knee replacement. If the surgeon is not vigilant in this regard, the patient will develop back pain relatively soon after the surgery depending on the size of the discrepancy. I have seen discrepancies up to 23 mm. This is totally unacceptable and must be avoided. In cases of small discrepancies (3mm – 12mm), heel lifts worn in the shoe may be used to level the pelvis. To correct extreme discrepancies, orthotic devices need to be built into the patient's shoe.

# Chapter Six

# Fibromyalgia

## Fibromyalgia Defined

No book for patients regarding back pain would be complete without the mention of fibromyalgia. This is an entity which involves muscles, tendons, ligaments, joints, and connective tissue. When this syndrome was first introduced many years ago, I had doubts regarding its true existence. However, over the years I've become convinced that this disease entity not only exists but also is extremely difficult to treat. It is probably overdiagnosed. I've seen many patients who have been saddled with the diagnosis of fibromyalgia who have a purely musculoskeletal dysfunction. This disease probably has its origins somewhere in the nervous system/brain. Fibromyalgia patients may be "wired" differently. It is not an entity which can be seen on any scan.

This disease seems to have components of both a collagen disorder and a muscular disorder. It occurs mostly in young women, although it may occur at any age and in either sex. Most of the patients report that they were healthy before they started having symptoms, having never had any type of back or joint pain. There is usually one incident that they can remember which activates the problem. The incident may be a simple one, not necessarily catastrophic. After that moment, they develop persistent pain which will not resolve. The intensity of the pain increases with time.

These patients complain of joint and muscle pain, continuous throughout the day and night, causing disruption in their sleep patterns. Sleep deprivation hinders their thinking process and intensifies the pain. The duration of the problem ultimately leads to depression. Most of these patients become overwhelmed by the pain and decrease their normal daily activities, thereby making the problem worse. The pain becomes the focus of their lives. The pain may disrupt their normal relationships with their spouses, families, co-workers, and friends. Their joints become stiffer and their muscles become weaker. They have a more difficult time performing normal activities both at home and at work. Some of these patients actually become disabled because of the disease process. Many become desperate, seeking out every imaginable therapy and test which a physician, nutritionist, chiropractor, physical therapist, acupuncturist, friend, or family member can recommend, hoping that a mistake was made in their diagnosis and they actually have a different disease process, preferably something curable. Some therapies may provide relief. Some are a waste of time where unscrupulous practitioners take advantage of these desperate people.

Are you sure you have it?

The process of diagnosing fibromyalgia is one of exclusion. The physician must rule out other diseases which mimic the symptoms with which you present. These tests will usually include comprehensive chemistry profiles, CBC, thyroid function tests, collagen profile tests, infectious disease testing, X-rays and possibly MRI/CT scans of involved joints, total body bone scans, and so on. You will be sent to multiple specialists including orthopedics, rheumatology, neurology, chiropractic, and sometimes infectious disease to leave no stone unturned. You undoubtedly will become more depressed during this workup since you will be told "everything is normal." Your hopes of finding a cure and resolving your problem once and for all usually result in disappointment, since very few therapies will satisfy your expectations. You lose confidence in physicians because they are definitely missing the cause of your problem. Typically, you refuse to accept the diagnosis of fibromyalgia without demanding other testing and consultation.

## Treatment protocols

I concentrate on three areas when I suspect a patient truly has fibromyalgia. I will never make this diagnosis on the first visit. Treatment strategy is spread over a few visits so I can assess what seems to work and what doesn't. Each patient with fibromyalgia is unique. There is not one treatment protocol that will work for every patient. I concentrate on restoring normal mechanics through osteopathic manipulation, provide analgesia for pain relief, and try to restore normal sleep patterns. Patients with fibromyalgia seem to manipulate much differently compared to musculoskeletal patients, more easily for the most part. I remember many times they manipulated so easily that I thought all their problems would resolve within the next forty-eight hours. In reality, these patients then call and complain that their pain has intensified. They seem to have a paradoxical response to manipulation compared to other patients who experience exceptional relief. Ice therapy, which works for many musculoskeletal problems, seems to aggravate their pain: many do better applying heat, as do rheumatoid arthritics. The response to NSAIDs (non-steroidal anti-inflammatory agents, such as ibuprofen) is variable. Some will get some relief, while others will get no relief whatsoever. They do get relief using analgesics. Because of the chronic intense pain which fibromyalgia patients suffer, they usually need narcotic medication for pain relief. This is fine if the patient is very conscientious and uses the medication judiciously. However, in reality many of these patients will escalate the prescribed dosages of short-acting narcotics and will become dependent on these medications. Some will need to be switched to long-acting narcotics to provide better control. Escalating the use of opioid narcotics may ultimately impair their judgment and coordination, further disrupt their sleep patterns, and worsen their depression. Non-narcotic analgesics, such as tramadol, may work in some patients. Antidepressant agents have been successful in helping restore sleep patterns and reduce depression. SSRI (serotonin reuptake inhibitor medications) and SNRI (serotonin-norepinephrine reuptake inhibitor medications) along with tricyclic antidepressants have been somewhat successful in controlling the depression and insomnia associated with fibromyalgia. Pregabalin (Lyrica) has recently become the only medication formally approved by the FDA for the treatment of fibromyalgia. This medication is a calcium channel modulator drug which inhibits the uptake of calcium ions in the nerve, keeping it from firing rapidly, decreasing excitation of the nerve, and causing a decrease in pain. Muscle relaxers also have shown some effectiveness in decreasing muscle spasticity. The drawback is they cause sedation and may affect coordination.


## Don't just sit around!

Exercise is probably one of the best treatments for this entity. Gentle stretching of the joints can be started and gradually increased to any exercise which you can tolerate and will perform regularly. Go for walks, get out of the house, socialize with neighbors and friends, swim, bicycle, whenever you are able. I find it very important that you try to stick to your routine as much as possible. This includes normal activities at home and at work. I want you never to develop a "disabled" mentality. If that happens, you will do very poorly. I want you to understand that you are not going to have good days every day of the week. No one does! Even on the bad days you need to push yourself to stay as close to "normal" as possible. You need the support of your family and friends to keep you functioning. You must keep pain-killers to a minimum and use them only when you truly need them. You must practice good sleep patterns, and not take naps throughout the day causing to you stay up all night. You must realize that many of these problems do stabilize over time. Consistency and motivation to succeed is the key to success! You may need psychological counseling to help you adapt to this life-altering situation. Family counseling is also a good idea since multiple members of the family may become stressed because of the change that is now occurring in everyone's lives due to this disease.

# Chapter Seven
# Osteopathic Medicine

When I was an undergraduate student at Loyola University in the early 1970's, the concept of Osteopathic Medicine was a well-kept secret. Everyone was competing to get into "medical schools." I became aware of this school of medicine when a close friend of mine, who was a year ahead of me in college, was accepted into their program. I had no knowledge of the concept of Osteopathic Medicine until it was explained to me by him, and then I scanned the course curriculum catalog. It seemed to be exactly like "medical school" with the addition of manipulative courses. What was spinal manipulation and for what was it used? What did it do? Why do it at all? The further I investigated this "new" school of medicine, the more comfortable I felt that I would learn skills and acquire abilities here that would not be possible in a typical M.D. (allopathic) school of medicine. I applied and was accepted in 1974. In my freshman year at the Chicago College of Osteopathic Medicine (CCOM), a course in the history of medicine, and osteopathic medicine in particular, was required. Since this was not a high-powered course on the way to becoming a physician, I along with many of my classmates felt this course to be a waste of our time. Today, I regret that such an attitude was prevalent. In order to know where you're going in your profession, it makes sense to know from where you came. Over the years patients have considered me their primary care physician. Most never differentiated between an allopathic (M.D.) versus an osteopathic (D.O.) physician. Many did not know the difference. All they knew is that I was there and helped them with their problems. They were not aware that for many years, early in my career, there existed discrimination against osteopathic physicians by the AMA, M.D.s, and their associated hospitals. With time, these barriers have been eroded. Doctors of Osteopathy now have all the same privileges and courtesies as are extended to their allopathic brethren. Many new osteopathic medical schools are being built, and the profession has grown very rapidly over the last hundred years. Osteopathic medicine encompasses every specialty and subspecialty available in allopathic medicine. The significant difference is our concept of biomechanics and the holistic approach upon which A.T Still founded osteopathic medicine.

A.T. Still was a physician who practiced in Kirksville, Missouri. I had always considered him just a "country doctor." I had never really thought about his true accomplishments until I visited Gettysburg on the way back from a convention in Washington D.C. some years ago. I was standing there with my family looking at the surgical tents with their instruments, crude by today's standards. Everything was geared up for amputating limbs. "How barbaric," I thought. Suddenly all the hairs on my arms stood up. So this was the medical profession in the era in which Dr. Still practiced. I could see why he felt he had a better way of meeting the needs of patients for whom therapies had not been far-reaching enough under conventional medicine. I no longer looked at him as a "country doctor," but now considered him a person far ahead of his time who had the courage to stand up against conventionalism and start his own medical profession. His philosophy was definitely a holistic medical approach. He felt there is an intimate relationship between the musculoskeletal system and the rest of the body, so much so that the musculoskeletal system reflects and interacts with the internal organs and vice versa. By considering both, you achieve a more effective treatment program for the patient.

The manipulative techniques Dr. Still developed are still in use today. Leaders in this profession have developed new techniques and have explored new concepts leading to deeper understanding of musculoskeletal mechanics, which have been made available to all osteopathic physicians. I've been in practice thirty years, and am still learning new techniques and approaches to help alleviate pain and suffering. Students always tell me they understand the theory of manipulative medicine, but are never able to experience its practical usage. In my office, they are able to get that experience. I do a lot of spinal manipulation in the office because I see a great number of mechanical problems which have not been resolved by other physicians.

The majority of these patients do very well. Their pain is alleviated. They need lower doses of medication for a shorter duration of time. The majority of patients with mechanical problems do not require surgery. For those who do require surgery, manipulation postoperatively at the appropriate time of healing can help restore function more quickly.

I also see a great deal of Family Practice-type cases in the office. Here, the students can see the difference between a true osteopathic physician and the conventional medicine of an allopathic physician. For example, imagine you have bronchitis and that you're coughing up yellowish-green sputum throughout the day and night. You have tightness in the chest. You feel short of breath. Breathing tests performed in the office show your small airways closing. Allopathic medicine may include a prescription for antibiotics, a cough suppressor, and possibly bronchodilator medicine. Osteopathic medicine will include all of those as well as manipulation to the chest, neck, and head which will improve breathing mechanics and lymphatic flow and make the drug treatment work more efficiently. You will feel better before leaving the office and will respond to the medical treatment faster and with fewer complications from the infection. Better mechanics in the chest wall with deeper breathing decrease the chances of developing pneumonia and collapsed lung.

What happens when you go to an M.D. complaining of headaches? You have tightness at the base of the skull, or all around your head. Your head feels as though it's in a vise. You are told that you have "muscle tension headaches." You are given medication, either a muscle relaxer or analgesic, to relieve the pain. In an osteopathic approach, medication may also be given, but manipulation to the upper thoracic spine, neck, and base of the skull is the primary treatment and will help to relieve the cause of the muscle tension which results in relief of the headache. Eliminating the cause of the problem eliminates the need for prolonged medication usage and prevents repeated attacks. Osteopathic physicians' therapy would also include a discussion on posture for both home and work situations which may be causing/aggravating the problem, and ways to correct it. A caution to keep in mind: unfortunately, in attempts to be accepted by our allopathic counterparts, some osteopathic physicians have either lost their manipulative skills or have never adequately developed them. As with any skill, all D.O.s are not created equal in regard to manipulative prowess, and unfortunately the results may vary from physician to physician.

# Chapter Eight
# Diagnostic Testing

This chapter is included to further describe the common testing ordered by physicians to investigate a diagnosis of back pain. I also give my opinions based on what I have seen in my years of practice as to the value each procedure has in determining treatment.

## X-Rays

What is seen on X-ray does not always correlate to back pain. They have limited value. If you took x-rays of one hundred people at random, you would probably find some pathology in almost all of them, depending on their ages and activities. Some will have back pain; others will not. Some of the worst-looking spines will show up in patients who have no pain whatsoever. Conversely, some of the best-looking spines will show up in patients who have constant back pain. This is because X-rays delineate anatomy. They cannot quantify function. A diagnosis of ruptured disc cannot be made from an X-ray. Disease can be suspected when narrowing of the disc spaces and intervertebral foramen are seen. The spinal cord and nerve roots do not show up on an X-ray. X-rays give an overview of spinal anatomy. They can show deformities that may not be able to be palpated. They can show abnormal curvature, either acquired or congenital. They may show metastatic disease. Think of an X-ray as a general map. It gets you to the general vicinity, but you need a more detailed inset to find the exact street for which you are looking.

## CT/MRI Scans

These scans are workhorses for evaluating the spine. CT scans sequence multiple X-rays, making numerous cuts through the spine to create a cross-sectional (side to side) image. The MRI uses a magnetic field to create similar images; however, it is also capable of making longitudinal (up and down) cuts in the spine which contribute more detail. Both use computers to create the images. These images can be highlighted to show even more detail. Sometimes contrast medium is used with the scans to enhance areas of great interest. They show the spine, spinal canal, exiting nerve roots, and so on. They are most useful in determining spinal canal stenosis (narrowing of the spinal canal enclosing the spinal cord), herniated discs, facet arthritis (inflammation in the joints connecting the vertebrae), inflammatory diseases, and spinal cord tumors. They are also utilized in evaluating the spine for recurrent symptoms and complications after surgery.

CT and MRI scans do not always correlate with back pain. Their best results occur when the pathology seen on the scan corresponds to physical findings and the patient's history. These scans do not necessarily tell if the problem is new or old unless serial scans have been performed over time and changes can be seen. Like any test, they show only one moment in time. If pathology is too small, it may not be seen on the scan. Serial scans performed over time may need to be performed if the problem does not resolve and the symptoms persist. As with X-rays, these scans show anatomy and do not necessarily reflect function. Surgical decisions should never be based solely on MRI or CT scans without a thorough evaluation of the patient and review of past treatments which have failed to resolve the problem.

## Bone Scans

These scans still have a place in evaluating the spine, although their role is somewhat limited compared to the one they played years ago. The patient is injected with a radioactive tracer which is absorbed into the bone and is read by a scanner. Images of the spine are limited to light and dark uptake of the radioactive tracer. Increased uptake is suspicious for possible metastatic disease (cancer) and acute inflammatory disorders (severe arthritis, infection). These scans show no cross-sectional images. I have found them to be especially effective in patients whose CT/MRI scans failed to show pathology but there was evidence that metastatic disease may have been present.

## Discograms

These studies are more invasive in nature. A surgeon or anesthesiologist injects contrast material, under sterile conditions, into the discs of the cervical or lumbar spine under pressure to see if he can duplicate the patient's pain patterns. If the pain is reproduced, the test is considered positive for that spinal level. This is not a routine test. It should be performed only when surgical intervention has been decided upon and there is still a question as to how many levels are involved in the pain mechanism.

## EMG (Electomyelogram)

These studies are usually performed by a neurologist. Needles are placed in the arms or legs and an electrical charge is applied. The nerve conduction velocity (the speed at which the nerve carries the electrical impulse) from one needle to the next is measured. A delay in the nerve conduction velocity would indicate some type of disease process either at the spinal cord level or in the nerve itself. The term "radiculopathy" means that the problem is stemming from the spinal cord level. The term "peripheral neuropathy" means that the problem is stemming from the nerve itself and is probably associated with some other metabolic disease such as diabetes, thyroid disease, or vitamin deficiencies.

The main drawback of this test is that it is not always positive when a disease process is present. It may not be sensitive enough to pick up early disease, even though the patient may already complain of symptoms. A negative test result does not mean that a disease process is not present, but that the instrument may not be sensitive enough to pick up the subtle changes that disease process is causing. A positive test indicates that some disease process is actively measurable. It is up to the physician to determine the cause of the problem, be it at the spinal cord level or in the nerve itself.

The EMG also measures muscle function. If the muscle does not respond as predicted to the electrical current, the test may show that there has been some damage to the muscle itself or to its nerve supply. It is imperative that the physician combine the information of the EMG with the patient's physical findings and history to make the proper interpretation and to determine the appropriate course of action. The EMG is most valuable in determining if multiple levels of the spine are involved in the pain mechanism or if the problem is originating from somewhere else entirely. For example, you complain of shoulder pain and have not responded to conservative therapy after an appropriate length of time. An MRI scan of your shoulder is performed and reveals some disease, which does not account for all of the pain you are suffering. An MRI scan of the cervical spine is then ordered to see if you are feeling referred pain to the shoulder. MRI shows some disease is present; however, it is not severe enough to explain all of your pain. The dilemma now exists: do we perform surgery to the shoulder, or to the neck, or will epidural injections to the cervical spine resolve the problem? A positive EMG in this circumstance would help to differentiate if the problem is coming from the cervical spine or from the shoulder so that appropriate therapy can be performed.

# Chapter Nine

# Surgical Options

## Epidural Injections

Epidural injections consist of a mixture of cortisone and a long-acting analgesic. These are administered by either an anesthesiologist or a surgeon into a space in the spinal canal called the epidural space. The patient can be either awake or asleep during the procedure. A fine needle is directed to the area of the pathology, where the medication is released. The areas of treatment are predetermined by evaluating MRI scans, examining the patient's physical findings, and listening to the pain pattern history. The needle is guided into the space using a type of X-ray machine called a fluoroscope. This is all done under sterile conditions.

The purpose of epidural injection is to concentrate anti-inflammatory medications at the site of the problem when oral medications have failed to have an effect. By reducing inflammation at the spine, or at the nerve roots leaving the spine, pain may be relieved. In order to appreciate the mechanism for this treatment, consider this example: Pretend that someone punches your arm as hard as he can. You will experience swelling, bruises, and pain. Some of this pain will radiate down into the forearm because of the muscular attachments and the way we lift and carry things throughout the day. That's what happened with disc disease at the spinal cord level. A disc has become weaker partially due to genetics and to normal wear and tear from activities of everyday life. At the right time in the right position and with the right force, that disc ruptures. The exploding force of that rupture allows the release of the inner softer disc material to hit the spinal cord or the nerve root, like the punch in the arm. The spinal cord/nerve root will swell and become inflamed at the area of the hit. This immediately will send signals from that level to higher areas of the spinal cord and brain. Signals will also be sent via the nerve root that is irritated to the back muscles innervated by that nerve. These muscles will tighten and redistribute the weight on the spinal column. All of this is instantaneous and automatic. All of this results in severe pain. Injecting this area with a cortisone/analgesic will in many instances help to calm down the trauma, alleviate pain, and decrease muscle spasticity.

Epidural injections are usually given in a series of three shots, a week or so apart. Be warned: patients do not always respond to the first injection. If you do, fantastic! If you don't, that doesn't mean that further shots will also fail. If the injections are done properly, at the right levels, some response should be seen by the second injection. If you combine this with osteopathic manipulative treatments you should get even better results. I have found in patients who respond to epidurals, there is a decrease in the amount of muscle spasm present in the back following successive injections. Patients usually go from being extremely tight in the area of the pathology to having the tissue become more normal in appearance and more pliable. Manipulation becomes easier to perform. Restoring normal spinal mechanics potentiates the effect of the epidural injection. You feel better and return to normal function using very few or no analgesics. Recovery time is faster with combination treatment than with epidural injections alone.

Some patients question the validity of doing epidural injections. They feel that we are only masking the pain and that the effect is only temporary. This is not true. The injections help to relieve inflammation. By doing this, they help to alleviate pain. The effect of the epidural injection can last indefinitely depending on the type of pathology and the willingness of the patient to follow instructions and to make lifestyle modifications which will prevent further damage to the disc/discs. Epidural injections may be extremely useful in patients with ruptured discs. They are somewhat less useful in patients with spinal stenosis, but definitely worth trying. They seem to have a higher failure rate in patients with far lateral herniated discs where the spinal nerve is pinned against the bony opening of the spinal column. They are absolutely a waste of time in patients with pure mechanical back or neck pain who fail to show pathology on the MRI scan, nor have they shown good results in fibromyalgia patients.

## A Word About Cortisone

Cortisone! With all the bad press about steroids nowadays, many patients are dead-set against taking this drug. They mistakenly associate it with "steroid usage" and refuse to consider using it. The truth regarding cortisone? Our bodies make this compound daily. The levels are higher in the morning and decrease toward evening. It is a natural compound which reacts to inflammatory and stressful states in our bodies. It is regulated by a thermostat-like region in the brain which controls the amount of cortisone produced each day for normal bodily functions. In patients with severe neck and low back pain, caused either by purely mechanical actions or by herniated disc, a short dosage of oral cortisone helps to relieve inflammation and makes it easier to manipulate and to respond to physical therapy compared to the use of non-steroidal anti-inflammatory medications, analgesics, or muscle relaxants. The cortisones are the strongest of the anti-inflammatory agents. Usually within three days I can see a decrease in muscle spasms and improvement in range of motion, allowing me to manipulate the same areas which were impossible to move prior to the use of the meds. Remember, the medication is a means to the cure, not the cure itself.

I have also noticed that the patients who exhibited a partial response to the oral cortisone but ultimately needed epidural injections always achieved better pain relief from the epidurals than did the cortisone non-responders. When one takes oral cortisone, the amount needed at the spinal level may not always be achievable. Here's what happens: the drug is consumed. It is then absorbed by the bowel, travels to the liver, then throughout the circulatory system. It eventually reaches the target at the spinal cord level, but is now at a dosage far smaller than that with which you started. Cortisone can be more tolerable in patients with sensitive stomachs or those who have peptic disease than non-steroidal anti-inflammatory agents. I've used cortisone in patients with peptic disease without any worsening of their symptoms for short periods of time.

This is the key: Prolonged use of oral cortisone suppresses the thermostat in the brain, decreases normal levels of cortisone production in the adrenal glands, and predisposes one to cataract formation, osteoporosis, and other medical entities. That is why we use a short course. Some patients complain of weight gain either from water retention or the urge to eat more while taking cortisone. I warn female patients that they might become more sentimental at higher dosages, while males might become more aggressive. These are all temporary side effects. The benefits of this medication definitely outweigh the potential side effects.

## Trigger Point Injections

In patients with acute or chronic back pain there occur areas in the muscles which become centers of activity that seem to keep the pain process going. There has been found to be electrochemical activity being generated from these centers. I describe this as a type of reflex that sets up between the receptors in the muscle and the spinal cord itself. Many patients will describe these "trigger point" areas as "knots" in the muscle. When they apply pressure to these areas they simultaneously feel pain and relief as well. Call it deep inhibitory pressure (in osteopathic manipulative lingo) or acupressure, the direct application of pressure to the most sensitive spot seems to calm the spot down in many instances. Now imagine using a needle with a syringe and injecting an anesthetic into those same areas. The trigger point is anesthetized, blocking the reflex that set up between that muscle and the spinal cord. Injecting these areas can provide relief which lasts indefinitely, especially when combined with manipulative treatment. I have seen a significant decrease in both the number and the intensity of the muscle spasms a week after trigger point injections which has allowed the patient to sleep better, exercise, and be manipulated more efficiently. Although trigger point injections are not effective in every patient, they have given relief to the majority of patients in whom I have used them. They do not seem to work so effectively in patients with fibromyalgia compared to those with other musculoskeletal problems.

## Microdiscectomy

For patients who have a ruptured disc with persistent back or neck pain and referred pain travelling down the arms or legs, and who have failed conservative therapy including manipulation, epidural injections, physical therapy, and oral medications, microscopic discectomy may provide relief. I stress, this is an elective procedure for patients who have failed all conservative therapies and are still symptomatic: nothing else has worked, and you're still in pain.

## In the Lower Back

In a lumbar microdiscectomy, after general anesthesia, an incision is made over the disc space which is involved in pain production. The overlying muscles are carefully separated away from the spinal column and a small window is created in the overlying bone of the spinal canal to allow access to the ruptured disc material and the spinal nerve. The extruded material is removed under direct observation with a microscope by careful dissection by the surgeon. The nerve root is then examined to make sure that there is no compression as it leaves the neurovertebral foramen. The bony defect (window) is covered with a fat pad removed from under the skin. The tissue layers are then sutured together. Recovery is relatively quick, after a short hospital stay. There is still support from the disc, which has been left in place. No spinal fusion was done. Sciatic pain resolves quickly if not immediately after surgery in a successful case.

## In the Neck

The cervical discs are much smaller than those found in the lumbar spine. With the patient under general anesthesia, the surgeon dissects to the damaged area. Decompressing the spinal cord and nerve root literally involves removal of the whole cervical disc. Techniques to stabilize the neck after surgery involve fusing the vertebrae above and below the removed disc with fragments of bone, and stabilizing these segments with a type of fixation device (plates and screws). The drawback is that some of these bony segments never fuse together to form one solid structure, and recovery may stretch over months to a year. Newer techniques involve the insertion of an artificial disc rather than cervical fusion. This may provide better stability and range of motion compared to cervical fusion, and the recovery period is shorter.

## Lumbar Laminectomy

This surgical technique is more appropriate for patients who are suffering from spinal stenosis. With the patient under general anesthesia, an incision is made encompassing the multiple vertebrae which are involved in creating the stenosis. The triangular-shaped portion on the spinal canal is carefully removed from all those vertebrae. The spinal nerves are decompressed. A fat layer is placed over the denuded spinal cord for protection. The tissue layers are then sutured closed. Time of recovery is lengthier compared to a microdiscectomy because of the multiple spinal levels involved. Patients may have more postoperative complications. Overall, when successful, the patient will have less pain extending down the legs.

## Lumbar Fusion

This procedure is controversial. The patient undergoes general anesthesia. The surgeon dissects down to the predetermined diseased discs. Discs that appear diseased on MRI or CT scans are removed in their entirety. Nerve roots are decompressed. The spaces left are filled with bone, cage devices, internal fixation devices (rods anchored to the bone), and recently, the artificial disc. Many of the patients who undergo this procedure are no better after and are maybe even worse than before they had the surgery. I do not recommend this procedure to my patients, nor do I refer to surgeons who routinely perform lumbar fusions for relief of back pain. The only indication for this procedure is to correct spondylolisthesis (slippage of one vertebra on the other) which has led to instability and possible spinal cord and nerve root compression, and is causing severe pain and/or a severely diseased disc which has not responded to any attempts to relieve pain. A disc replacement may be beneficial. In my experience, surgeons who promote spinal fusions have a tendency to perform more surgery than is necessary. Their outcomes may be beneficial in some patients. However, I've not seen this to be the case in the majority of the patients I have seen post-op in my practice. Many of these patients must rely on permanent pain management, using narcotics for the rest of their lives. Others may undergo multiple surgeries because their pain did not subside after the first procedure. This disrupts more of the spinal anatomy, leading to further instability and unfortunately increased pain.

## Percutaneous Techniques

Pain can sometimes be generated strictly by the disc itself. The approach to alleviating this type of pain may involve trying to destroy the nerve supply to the pain-generating disc itself. One procedure involves intradiskal heating (IDET) in which a small wire is introduced into the posterior portion of the disc. The nerve supply is heated and destroyed. This technique does not benefit all patients. In the proper hands, with the appropriate patient, beneficial results may be obtained.

There are other techniques which have been used percutaneously to relieve disc pain. Some involve injection of corticosteroids into the disc. Some involve extraction of the disc via mechanical or laser devices. The most important point to remember is that each of these procedures has very strict criteria to insure that the patient is appropriate for that procedure and will obtain the best result. If the original criteria are not followed to the letter by the surgeon, the results may not be good. The patient should be thoroughly evaluated by the surgeon. All information about previous therapies, both successes and failures, should be discussed and taken into consideration along with all of the diagnostic testing to determine if those prior procedures had a chance to work and if the patient meets all the presurgical criteria for this procedure. Failure to fulfill the strict criteria set by the pioneers of these techniques may be one of the reasons why patients who undergo repeated surgeries have poor outcomes. Care must be taken to insure that this patient has failed all conservative measures before undergoing any aggressive therapy.

Facet Injections

The facets of the vertebra are small angular cuts on its bony surface. They connect with similar ones on the vertebra above and below them and form synovial joints (joints similar to the ones in your fingers, toes, knees but much smaller). Just as your fingers or knees can become irritated from trauma or arthritis, so can these joints in your spinal column. In patients with facet pain, cortisone/anesthetic agents are injected into the facet joints under fluoroscopy by a surgeon or anesthesiologist. This technique has been successful in relieving back pain caused by these irritated facets.

# Chapter Ten

# The Do's and Don'ts of Neck and Back Pain

As you have seen, there is no one solution for everyone's neck and back pain. We are all individuals. We all (with the possible exception of identical twins) have different genetic codes, physical susceptibilities, pain thresholds, recovery rates, occupations, pastimes, hobbies/sports, and so on. To say there is only one way to recover from back pain is foolish and misleading. There are, however, basic concepts that everyone can follow which will give some relief and control over these problems.

Don't become depressed over the fact that you seem to have no control over your pain. First of all, you need to be realistic. Just because you can't achieve 100% relief doesn't mean that you or your doctors have failed. Some relief and improved mobility is better than nothing at all. The question is, how far are you willing to go to achieve more relief?

Secondly, if you truly feel that taking a pill is going to solve all of your problems, you probably are mistaken. As I have tried to stress in these pages, drugs are a means to an end, not the end in themselves. The potential for addiction is low; however, it does exist.

The following are instructions and advice which I give to all my back pain patients. They have already been mentioned in various previous chapters, but I thought it would be good to list them all again in one place for you to reference when needed.

## #1   Cold Packs

In an acute injury or an aggravation of a pre-existing back problem, you're always safe using ice. The ice prevents congestion and protects already irritated muscles or muscle groups from becoming waterlogged and suffering more intense spasm. The ice pack should cover the areas of the back that are feeling the pain. In areas with referred pain such as the arms or legs, the ice pack should be placed on the neck or lower back. Don't apply the ice pack to the areas in the extremities where you feel the referred pain, because that's not the area from which the pain is originating. Do not apply the ice pack directly to the skin. Use the ice pack over clothing or a towel until the ice melts. Do NOT alternate cold with heat.

Any form of ice can be used. Refreezable gel packs are pliable and last a reasonably long period of time. Patients have had success using ice cubes in plastic bags, or even bags of frozen vegetables. There's no specific length of time for icing—use as much as you want, for as long as you are comfortable. You may find applying an ice pack to the back will help alleviate pain and allow you to sleep better. If you are going to experience prolonged driving time when getting to work or going on an extended trip, try applying gel packs to your back when driving or sitting in the car. Spare gel packs can be kept cold in a cooler to change when necessary.

## #2   Heat Application

Patients who have advanced osteoarthritis seem to do better with moist heat applications than they do with ice packs. This is also true for patients with underlying collagen diseases such as rheumatoid arthritis, systemic lupus, or fibromyalgia. Heat can be in the form of a hot bathtub, whirlpool, or moist heating pad set on low. Again, there is no time limit to the heat you can apply. Please use common sense with regard to your overall physical condition and pre-existing medical problems. Check with your physician to make sure you will not make your cardiovascular disease or other medical problems worse with heat applications. Twenty minutes for a hot bath or whirlpool soak may be appropriate for most patients. Never fall asleep using a heating pad, since serious burns can develop.

## #3   Posture

Good posture is extremely important in helping to keep back pain under control.

- Mother knew best: Stand up straight! Do not slouch. When standing, do not shift your weight from one side to the other, but carry your weight balanced over your right and left legs equally.
- Do not read or watch TV in bed propped up with pillows. Don't lie on the sofa with your head propped up on your arm watching TV, reading, or listening to music.
- Sit on a firm chair with a small pillow or cushion placed in the small of the back (lumbar spine).
- When driving or sitting in the car, push your buttocks as far back in the seat as possible, with the small pillow behind your low back. Then buckle your seat belt and shoulder harness. This will pull you tightly into the seat and promote good sitting posture for the lumbar spine and the neck. If you have lumbar supports built into your car seats, adjust them to give maximum support.
- When working at the computer, adjust your work station to allow you to look directly at the monitor. You should be sitting upright with your head balanced over your shoulders, not looking to the right or to the left for prolonged periods. Place your laptop on a surface other than your lap if you will be working for a long period. It needs to be at the correct height to avoid forward bending your head to look at the screen for long periods of time.
- If you need to use the telephone throughout the day, wear a headset. Do not cup the telephone handset between your head and shoulder.
- Whatever you are doing, be it sitting at the computer, reading, knitting or crocheting, watching TV, driving or riding in a vehicle or aircraft, periodically get up and walk around. Take small breaks to stretch your neck, shoulders, and back. Do not stay in the same position for long periods of time.
- If you are in an occupation which requires heavy lifting or getting into very cramped spaces, avoid forward bending at the waist. Lift with your arms and legs. Keep your back as straight as possible. The thrust needed to lift a heavy object when bending forward and slightly off-balance can initiate or

aggravate back pain. Use any tool you can obtain to provide a mechanical advantage and avoid injuring your back or neck. If it takes two people to lift an object, don't attempt it by yourself—get help!

- If your back does go into spasm, move slowly. Quick, sudden moves will cause the spasm to intensify and increased pain will be the result. Try to stretch your back or neck out slowly, moving into extension. Remember, discs rupture in a flexed position, not in extension.

## #4  Heel Lifts

If you have been diagnosed with Unequal Leg Length Syndrome, and a heel lift has been prescribed, you must wear it at all time when up and walking about. Do not complain of recurrent back pain if you are not wearing your heel lift in all your pairs of shoes, at work and at home. During the summer months, flip-flop wearers neglect their heel lifts, and as a consequence suffer back pain. Not wearing the heel lift allows the instability in your back to go unequalized, and that instability will translate into back and neck pain. You have no one to blame but yourself when you neglect to use this simple device to balance your pelvis.

The heel lift should be the appropriate thickness to level the pelvis. You will experience greater low back, hip and sometimes even knee pain if the lift is too thick. Vice versa, you may experience a persistence of pain if the lift is too thin. The thickness that balances out your short leg and creates a level pelvis is the one that is just right.

## #5  Sleep Posture

The most neutral position when sleeping is sleeping on your side. Right or left does not matter and is a personal preference. You should not sleep in a fetal position with your knees drawn up to your chest. This may stimulate the prevertebral muscles involved in lower back pain, causing them to tighten during the night and resulting in your feeling severe stiffness in the morning upon rising. Place a small pillow between your knees to help keep your legs level with your pelvis. This will help decrease pain in the lower back and hip region.

Turning over in bed will sometimes wake you up and aggravate pain. If this should occur, get out of bed and walk and stretch gently. You'll get back to sleep much more quickly than by just lying there or by tossing and turning trying to find a new comfortable position.

Use only one pillow when sleeping. Try to keep your neck and head in a neutral position preventing excessive flexion/extension or lateral flexion (side-bending). Sleeping on two or more pillows puts your neck in that position of extreme flexion or side-bending, and promotes increased muscle tension.

Do not read or watch TV in bed. Do not allow your head to snap forward or backward while you are trying to stay awake watching television. Jerking the head forward and back acts like small whiplash injuries and aggravates the neck and upper back. Do not fall asleep on the couch watching TV. Wake up and go to bed!

## #6 Exercising: Low Back

Exercising and stretching are extremely important in preventing and controlling low back pain. Exercise activity depends on your age, physical condition, and concomitant medical problems/disabilities. It is important to avoid exercises which involve flexion in the low back. DO NOT DO toe touches, sit-ups, or bringing your knees up to your chest. Flexion exerts an extreme amount of force in the lower lumbar spine. If you have ruptured a disc or have an injured disc that is about to rupture, these maneuvers will aggravate the problem.

You cannot go wrong using extension exercises in the lower back. You cannot rupture a disc or fracture vertebrae (in cases of osteoporosis/ osteopenia) in extension (backward bending).

An easy exercise to accomplish extension is as follows:
- Roll up a towel in the shape of a log from 4" to 6" in diameter. The roll can be secured with rubber bands. The tighter and firmer the roll, the more force it will exert on the lumbar spine in extension. ( Figure 10.1)

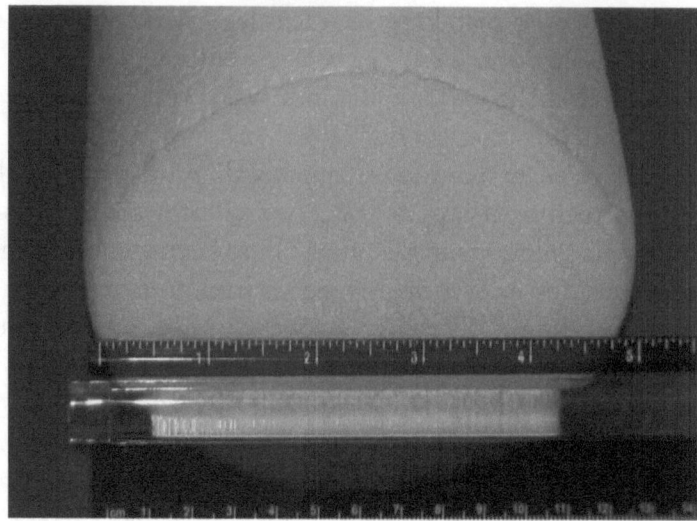

Figure 10.1 5" diameter Roll

- Lie down on the floor and place the roll under your back crosswise to the spine at the bottom of your ribcage. As you lie on the roll, it will act as a fulcrum stretching the back. The muscles in front of the spine will start to contract and try to pull you off the roll. You will feel tightness in the lower back, in proportion to the amount of muscle spasm. If your back is extremely tight, lying on the roll may feel unbearable, and your back will not extend. In that case, just lying flat on the floor may provide some relief. (Figure 10.2)

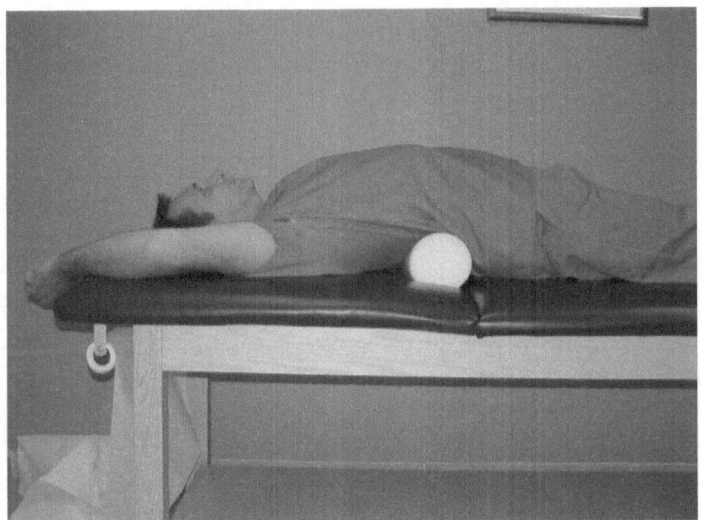

Figure 10.2 Roll at the bottom of the Ribcage

- After a few minutes, the muscles in front of the spine will begin to fatigue. This will allow your lower back to reach full extension.
- Do this exercise as many times a day as you would like. You need lie on the roll only for a few minutes at a time.
- If you are elderly or afraid to lie on the floor, you can accomplish the same thing by making the roll bigger and lying on the bed.

**CAUTION: If you have had previous back surgery involving the placement of fixation devices such as rods or plates, these exercises may not be possible for you to do. Discuss these with your physician/surgeon before starting them to see if they will cause any complications regarding your previous surgery.**

Another way to extend your lower back is with the following exercise:
- Lie flat on your belly on the floor or bed.
- At the same time, lift your right arm straight out in front of you and your left leg off the floor a few inches. Hold for two counts. (Figure 10.3)

- Alternate each arm-leg combination. Aim for five times with each combination, increasing the hold time to five counts as you become able.

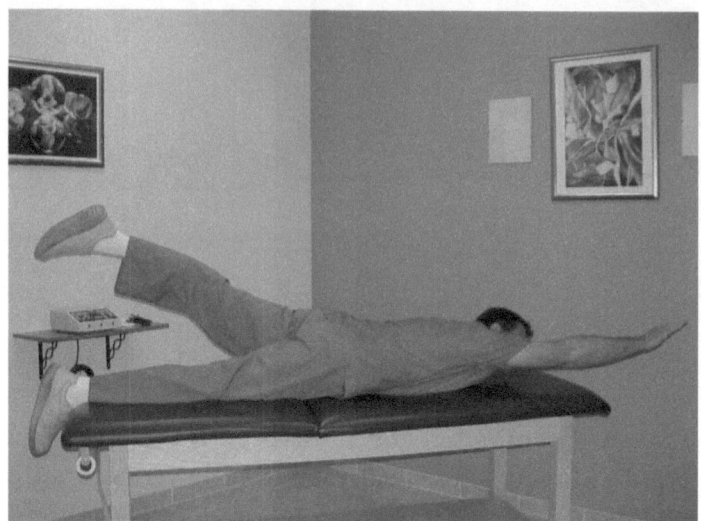

Figure 10.3  Arm/Leg Lifts

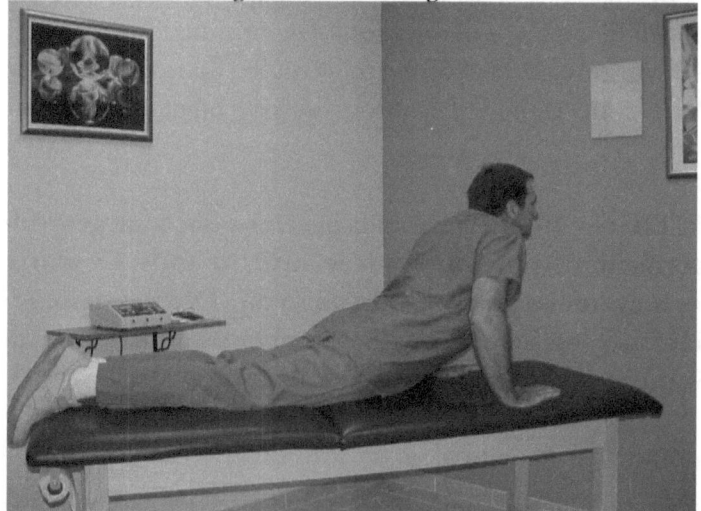

Figure 10.4  Cobra Pose

A Yoga Pose sometimes known as the Cobra is a good extension exercise:

- Lie flat on your belly on the floor or bed.

- Raise your upper body off the floor, supporting yourself on your hands as though doing a push-up (Figure 10.4).
- Hold for two counts.
- Lower yourself slowly to the starting position.
- Do as many reps up to five, increasing the time held as you are able.

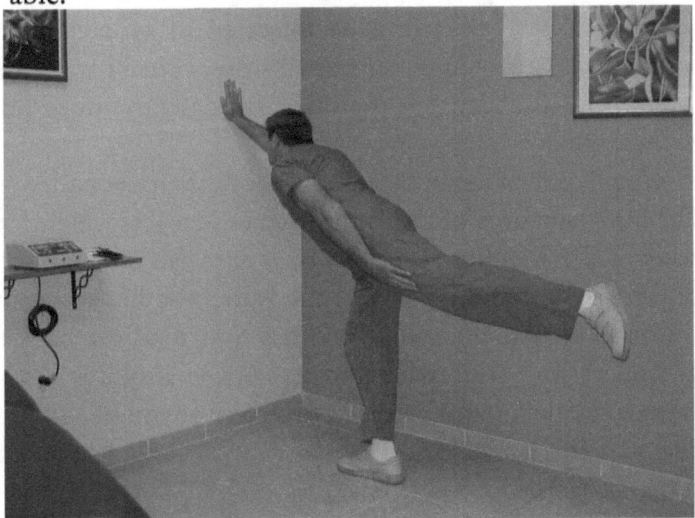

Figure 10.5 Wall Stretch

Another gentle stretching exercise:
- While facing a wall, rest one hand against it.
- Now extend the leg on the opposite side, leaning toward the wall, keeping the knee straight. Hold for two counts. (Figure 10.5)
- Now alternate the hand-leg combination. Aim for five times with each combination at the beginning. You may increase the reps as you become able.

**If you have any questions as to your ability to perform these exercises, discuss them with your physician or surgeon before attempting them.**

Bicycling, either on a conventional bike or a stationary bike, does seem to help alleviate low back pain. You should sit up straight while riding. Sitting in a flexed position hunched over the handlebars will defeat the purpose of this exercise. The prevertebral muscles in the lower lumbar spine attach to the front of both thighs. The alternating flexion/extension of the thigh muscles while pedaling may fatigue the tight flexor muscles and relieve lower back spasm. If you have arthritic knees, adjust the seat to a higher level to allow you to exercise without creating knee pain. When using a conventional bike, ride on a level surface. With any biking exercise, start slowly for ten to fifteen minutes and gradually increase your time as tolerated in proportion to your health status. Again, if you have heart disease, consult your physician before attempting any vigorous exercise, especially in hot or otherwise inclement weather.

Swimming is one of the best exercises for both upper and lower back pain. The buoyant force of the water makes you feel weightless. It is much easier to do stretching exercises in water than on land because of that very fact. The cooling effect of the water also has some analgesic effect. In order to actually swim, one has to extend the back to keep from sinking. Using your arms and legs while stroking and kicking exercises both the flexor and extensor muscles. If you like to jog, using a flotation vest in the deep end of the pool will allow you to do so without aggravating your lower back.

Exercises to avoid while you are in the acute phase of low back pain include weightlifting. Once stable, you may lift weights so long as you do not attempt to lift more than your capabilities. You must be extremely careful with free weights to avoid being pulled off balance when lifting. Jogging should also not be performed in the acute phase of low back pain. The repetitive bouncing action in the pelvis will aggravate low back pain. You are encouraged to walk, and avoid prolonged sitting or inactivity.

If you're concerned about losing tone while you are having back pain, you can substitute leg lifts and mild crunches in place of your flexion exercises to tighten up your abdominal muscles:

- Lie flat on your back and bring your legs up together slowly. You will feel tightness in the thigh muscles first.
- Raising the legs higher will be felt in the pelvis, and finally in the abdomen.
- Hold in the position where the abdominal muscles are tightening for a few slow counts. (Figure 10.6)
- Slowly bring the legs back to the ground.

- Repeat as many times as desired.

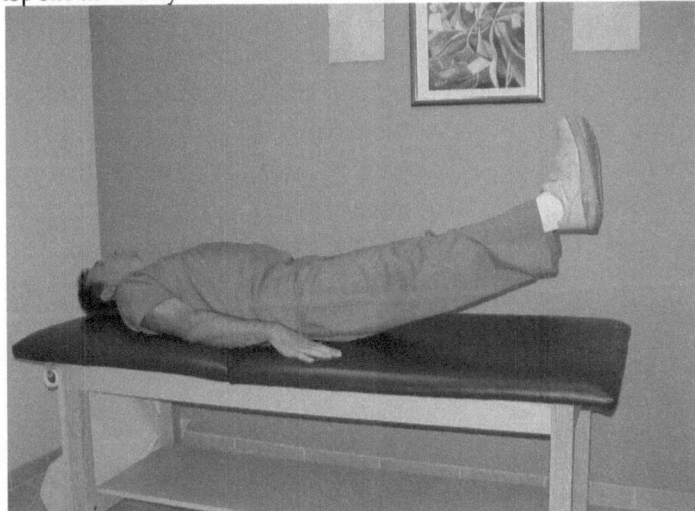

Figure 10.6 Leg Lifts

Mild crunches can be accomplished by

- lying flat on your back, then turning slightly on one side.
- Flex your head and upper body GENTLY until tightness is felt in the abdominal muscles. (Figure 10.7)

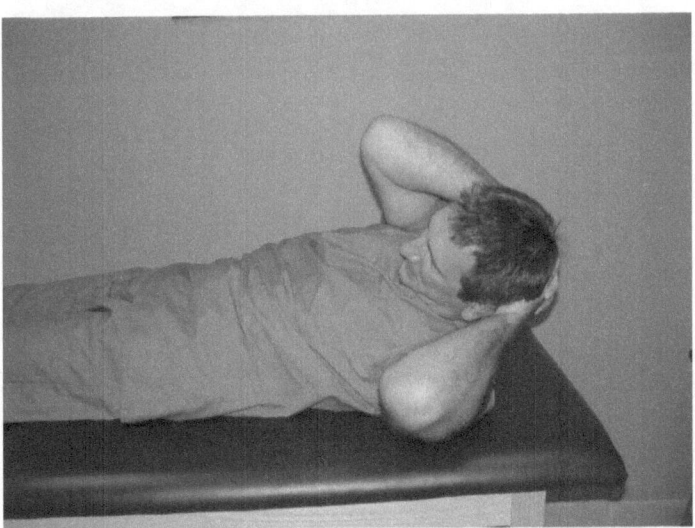

Figure 10.7 Mild Crunches

- Turn on the other side and repeat as many times as desired, alternating sides.

## #7  Exercising: Upper Back

I have not found a lot of exercises that are good for stretching the upper back. When you have neck pain, in acute spasm, you do not want to move your neck or turn your head. You feel as though your head weighs 1000 pounds and any little movement creates a surge of pain. Gentle range of motion exercises including mild extension and rotation to each side (Figure 10.8), and side-bending to the right and left (Figures 10.9 and 10.10) are necessary to relieve muscle spasm.

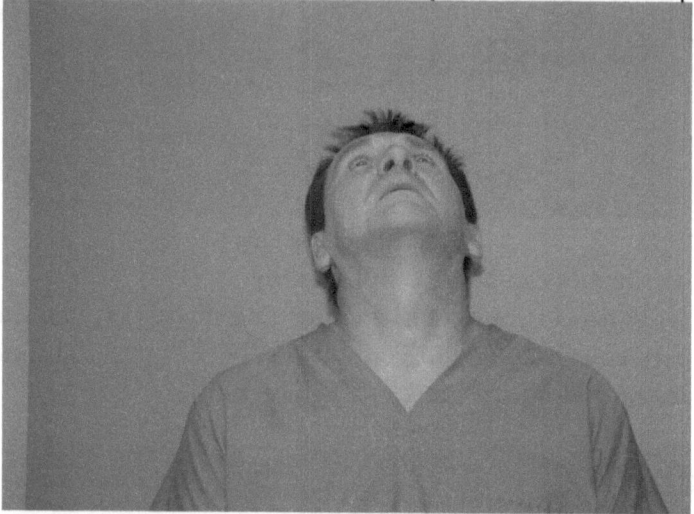

Figure 10.8  Extend the Head, then rotate it around in a circle

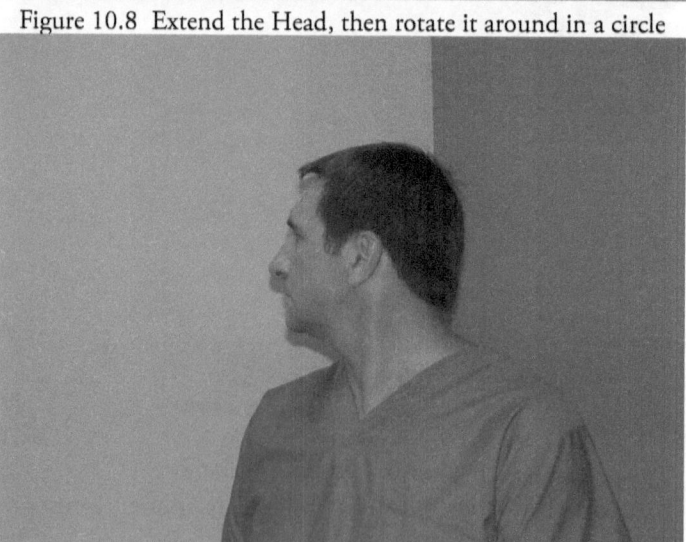

Figure 10.9  Side-bending to the Right

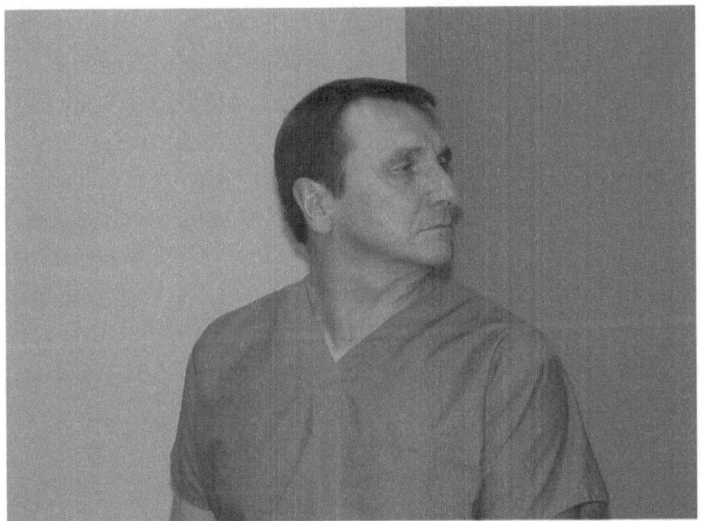

Figure 10.10 Side-bending to the Left

If you have a history of flattening of the cervical spine, try this variation of the rolled-up towel exercise for the low back mentioned in a previous chapter:

- Roll up a towel to reach a one- to two-inch diameter
- Lie down on the floor and place the towel roll behind your neck, letting the neck slowly stretch to the extent of the roll.
- If you lie on a bed instead of the floor, the diameter of the roll needs to be increased. If you experience any choking or neck pressure, the roll must be made smaller. To get some extension at the base of the shoulders, the roll should be a diameter of two- to four- inches.
- Lie on the roll for a few minutes as many times a day as tolerated.

Swimming is also a good exercise to stretch the neck, upper back, and shoulders. It may help provide increased mobility and decreased muscle spasm and pain. Weightlifting should be avoided during acute neck and upper back spasms. It may be used after you are stable if you so desire. **Again, previous surgeries may prohibit you from performing the above exercises, and you must clear them with your physician before starting any exercise program.**

## #8   Medications

By now, you know my philosophy on medication: it does have a place in the treatment of acute and chronic upper and lower back pain. You must follow your doctor's instructions to the letter and use the medications only as prescribed. The medication is a means to an end rather than the end itself. You should always be on guard to avoid becoming dependent on narcotic analgesics. Do not anticipate pain, but use the appropriate analgesics only when necessary to provide pain relief. Never accelerate the use of narcotics just to be able to perform additional activities which may be aggravating your neck and lower back pain.

## #9   Weight Reduction

Some physicians use the excuse that your back problems are caused by your excessive weight, and unless you reach normal weight you will never get better. You should strive to reach and stay at ideal body weight to keep yourself healthy. Obesity creates insulin resistance, which leads to diabetes and heart disease. But your back pain will not magically disappear once you reach ideal body weight. Weight does play a role in low back pain; however, it has been my experience that you can get better even if you don't lose any weight, depending on what caused your back pain. The fact that you may be obese is a poor excuse to explain why you can't get relief of low back or neck pain.

## #10   Activities

You must realize that the human body was not designed to perform certain activities, and that your insistence on the performance of those activities when you're healthy might have to be modified when you are not. Contact sports, outdoor activities, or indoor projects that aggravate your back pain will have to be curtailed while you are in the acute phase, if you are interested at all in recovery. Taking an extra dose of narcotics so that you can get through the activity is detrimental to your overall health and well-being. If your job is causing you to have chronic back pain, seriously consider changing jobs.

# Chapter Eleven
# Choosing a Surgeon

## When All Else Fails....

Choosing a back surgeon by looking in the phonebook and being drawn in by the most enticing ad is probably not a good plan. Neither is grabbing the most popular one in town because of a lavish TV spot. Presumably, your primary care physician has been working with you up to this point. Conservative therapy has failed. Pathology seen on MRI or CT scans or other tests matches your physical findings. You and your primary care physician feel that you're now a surgical candidate.

Usually, your primary care physician has some working relationship with either a neurosurgeon or an orthopedic surgeon specializing in backs to whom patients have been referred. Preferably those patients have had successful outcomes. The recommendation to a particular surgeon should be based on the type of problem you have and the expertise of that particular surgeon for that particular problem.

All surgeons are not necessarily equal in abilities, skills, and experience. Some far surpass others. Good surgeons do a thorough physical examination, take time to listen to you, take into consideration all therapy performed so far, carefully examine any previous scans, and decide if any other conservative measure may be appropriate before scheduling surgery. All your questions should be answered. If surgical intervention is deemed necessary, the least invasive procedure to get the job done should be recommended. If the surgeon is unwilling to sit and discuss the ramifications of the procedure with you, get a second opinion. Sometimes that needs to be done outside your own community. If the surgeon is unwilling to take the time with you beforehand, how can you feel comfortable about the aftercare, or trust that there will be support in case complications occur or your expectations are not met?

Surgery should be your last resort. Make sure that you find the right surgeon with whom you feel comfortable and in whose abilities you have confidence.

# Chapter Twelve
# In Conclusion

Suffering back pain can be very debilitating and depressing. It is sometimes overwhelming to both the patient and the family. It can alter relationships, destroy careers, and create disabilities both temporary and permanent. The purpose of this book was to try to give you the patient an understanding of the causes, diagnosis, treatment, and complications of back problems. It was written to emphasize that you can gain control over this disease process. It is not hopeless!

Contrary to what you may have been told, you do not have to live your entire life in pain. Many of the solutions to this problem may be rather simple. Often they are overlooked because we focus on high-tech solutions to relatively simple problems. Reliance on drug therapy for "happily ever after" is naïve and unrealistic.

In these pages I've attempted to delineate the alternative approaches to treating neck and back pain which have served my patients well for thirty years. Conservative therapy has been successful in treating the vast majority of patients with back pain. Osteopathic manipulation and epidural injections have enabled most to avoid surgery.

Common sense and a willingness to make some lifestyle modifications are the keys to controlling flare-ups of back pain. You must be willing to work to get back to normal, and continue to work to stay normal, even if you do require surgery. Never adopt a "disabled" mentality. Force yourself to exercise even if it is uncomfortable at first. Depression associated with pain must be treated appropriately with antidepressant agents. Sleep disorders can be corrected.

Success may come easily for some people. For others, like those who suffer from fibromyalgia, it will be an uphill battle. Your condition will not be resolved by popping a pill, or by a handful of pills. It may involve giving up doing something you truly love. It may require changing an occupation to one which is more compatible with what you are capable of doing without aggravating pain. You must be willing to take responsibility for your health and well-being. When you can commit to a lifelong venture of acceptance of your physical limitations, and you resolve to make the best of your remaining abilities, you will achieve success.

www.ingramcontent.com/pod-product-compliance
Lightning Source LLC
Chambersburg PA
CBHW031258280526
45784CB00004B/1896